Your Feelings

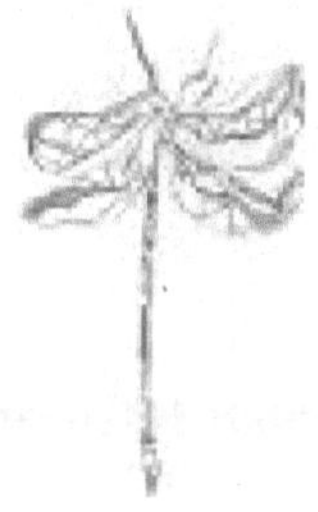

Bad news: You can't control anything but your thoughts. The good news is that you can control everything with your thoughts.

–Debasish Mridha

How can we allow the devastating news to be shared without being crushed or imprisoned? How can we make the next step, unimaginable but necessary, towards God knows what? How can we find peace of heart?

When there is no peace within us?

Even when you are in an "oh my God", you can still acknowledge that your mind can control you. Even when events happen beyond our control, we have the power to make conscious decisions and ask powerful questions like: What do I do with this situation?

This idea is not for you. Think about times when one crisis came after another. The first thing disappeared and the second became huge.

A friend of mine says to me, "Never say it cannot get worse, because it always can!" I disagree. It can always get better.

Let me show you an example. It was a horrible day. It was the worst I could imagine, and it was so hard to separate my thoughts from it. I was stuck in the "worrying about it" stage for hours. It was then that something unexpected happened. My thoughts and emotions were now focused on something completely different. Where were the old feelings? Why do these obsessive, huge feelings seem so small?

You will notice your emotions rise and then fade as you pay more attention. They can almost overwhelm you. They then recede around you. What can you do to let them rise and then fall without taking you out on the open seas?

Be careful before you start to say "I can't do this!" This can change easily from "This is terrible" to "OK. We can overcome this challenge and be more successful at the end."?

How might something better be true? What might be some alternative thought, one that will give you hope? Even if it is outrageous, ask, "what if...?"

CHAPTER ONE

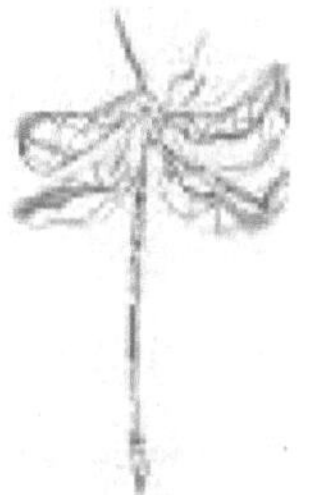

Not Like Any Other Day

It's amazing how your worst day often begins exactly like every other. It's possible to complain about it all silently to yourself. It's possible to wish for something more, to break from the routine. Just when you feel you can't take it anymore, something happens that makes you wish your day wasn't so boring.

–Joanna Cannon

January 1, 2015, was Sunday. It was the first day in Dubai. I was always F the first to get up, as usual. I moved slowly so Samer wouldn't wake me, while I did my hair and makeup and then got into my gym clothes. My first Jumeirah client was on a strength training session. My nine-year old son was ready to go before I set out to work. I crept into Yousef's bedroom and pulled the curtains aside. I reached into the bunk bed of Yousef and kissed him. I didn't know it would be the last time this would happen.

"Good morning, Yousef! It's time to get up!" I replied.

When he's still asleep, he looks so adorable in the morning. He was not fussy and got dressed in his white and purple shirt and navy blue shorts with socks.

My Swedish coffee was ready to go in the kitchen. I waited for Yousef and then I had a glass of lemon water. I also ate a banana thinking about how fortunate I was to have my first client make me a sandwich after I trained with them.

Yousef was eating his cereal while I looked out of my living room window. The Sheikh Zayed Road was still very busy, but there wasn't much traffic. Dubai is one the most cosmopolitan and cosmopolitan places in the world. It is constantly changing, growing and becoming more congested. It's a beautiful location near the beach and the desert. It is "hot like an oven with lots of buildings everywhere you go," Yousef says. Dubai has every luxury brand, designer store, and international restaurant. There's also a mix of expats from around the globe. I lived in between two metro stations and watched the train go by. This scene is a picture of my past life, and it's what I remember.

I dropped Yousef at school before eight o'clock and began walking through the beautiful garden of my client, which was full of palm, orange, and fragrant flowers on my way to my elegant home. She smiled as usual, and she walked down the stairs to her private gym at 8:20 a.m. It was a blessing to have worked with such a kind and generous woman. It was a wonderful way to live my life.

Before I left for home, Samer helped me to make cosa, Yousef’s favorite dish. Samer took out the middle of the small zucchini and I filled it with minced meat, rice, and other ingredients. We all love to cook and eat healthy food, particularly Lebanese, which is my favorite. It used to be something I did all the time. But now, these little rituals are precious memories.

Yousef loved football and played after school every day. He was usually at my house by 2.30 on Sundays, but I received a call that day.

"Helene! It's Suzy! You have to get down to the school immediately!

Yousef may have broken his leg when he injured it.

"What happened?" I asked. Alarm bells started ringing in my head.

She said, "He was running and then he fell and started screaming.". This was what I tried to do. It was a fall, wasn't it? It happens all the while in soccer.

"The nurse advised him not to move his leg. Suzy asked, "Should we call the ambulance?".

I replied, "Let's call his dad!".

Samer was driving the car and picked up the phone right away. He was right there, so he ran over to the school before me. I ran downstairs to hail a taxi. It is amazing that when you need something urgently, it is so difficult to get hold of it. It could just be that it is.

Finally, I got in a taxi and asked the driver to take me to Rashid Hospital as quickly as possible. It was unbelievable to me that he made a wrong turn and drove in the opposite direction. Anxious, frustrated, and anxious, I finally arrived at the hospital and found Yousef in a wheelchair looking lost and worried.

They put Yousef's leg in a cast, and informed us that he would be out of school for six more weeks. I took a photo of Yousef looking dejected. He was obviously in pain and unhappy that he would not be playing football for how many weeks. He looks much better in the picture the next day. His leg is still sticking out and he was cheered by Laith's Nerf gun.

I was most concerned about contacting his teachers to ask them for help with homework. Lynn, the school nurse, was also my concern. I thought about the classes he would miss and wondered how I would wash him. All the details of a child with a broken leg kept me busy. He was on a school holiday, so he wouldn't have to miss school as much. It wasn't long before Yousef was getting around on his crutches and we were able take him out for a bit.

Three weeks later, Yousef was feeling very trapped and ready to go back to school. He invited Mo, his friend, over to play. Then, Yousef started screaming. I ran to his room and found him on the ground. Although I assumed they were jumping or doing something, Mo told me that Yousef had tripped on his crutches. Mo stood there in horror, staring at Yousef scream on the ground. His panic and pain seemed exaggerated. He seemed to be mostly afraid since the fall wasn't too severe. Although he was still crying, I tried to calm him down. Mo returned home and I called a friend, who informed me of a homeopathic pain medication, which the pharmacy delivered. It didn't work for Yousef. I

Could not understand his strong reaction when he fell. He wouldn't have broken his leg twice - anyone ever heard of it? A cast is required to break a leg?

We took him to the hospital because he was still in pain the previous night. He was then x-rayed. The ER doctor confirmed that it had fractured again. Samer and me both saw something wrong with the xray. It wasn't a clear break. We knew something was wrong, but we didn't know what it was. We didn't know what we knew. It was that afternoon that I received a call from a different doctor. He explained that he had been reviewing the x-rays and found something that the doctor from the ER hadn't noticed.

He assured us that there was nothing to worry about and recommended that I take Yousef to the hospital to have his leg examined. Samer was out of town by this point. However, when I called him and explained what the doctor had said, he invited a friend to accompany me to the ER, where Wesef was admitted. He had blood tests on Monday and a CT scan of the leg. He stayed at the hospital overnight.

Our lives were forever changed on Tuesday morning. My memory of standing in the hallway at Rashid Hospital and listening to my son's doctors tell me that he had cancer will be etched in my heart forever. It was Ewing's Sarcoma, they suspected. "What's that?" I asked.

"Cancer of the bone."

These men were telling me that my son had bone disease?

Two doctors left and one stayed to continue talking. He suggested they could perform a biopsy in another Dubai hospital. He advised me the next thing.

He said, "Go back to the country.".

Although I'm Swedish, I have lived in Dubai for more than 25 years. Was he referring to Dubai? Dubai was my home.

"Is it because you're afraid that it will spread?" I inquired.

He explained that it was a rare form of cancer and needed a special operation.

He said, "They don't have specialists here to treat children's cancer.".

I asked him, "Do you have any children?" He answered yes. He said, "Where would your child go?" "Germany," he replied.

Did I hear him right? Did he tell me to leave my house? And where are you going?

Sweden or Germany? I was thinking about Yousef's malignant tumor. I wanted to find out if it was cancer and at what stage. Is it spreading? It was spreading. I was overwhelmed with questions and turmoil. My child was in another place and had no idea what was happening. What would I say to him?

The doctor's voice faded as thoughts came and went. Everything around me sounded muffled. I felt detached from the world and disconnected, almost as though I was watching it from afar. I finally turned my back on the doctor and focused on the door at the end the long corridor. I continued walking down the endless hallway, noting out of my corner that the walls were moving in front of me. Finally, I opened the door at the end and walked down the stairs in a trance. It was all a dream.

Yoursef's father was still at work, at an exhibition held in Doha, Qatar. His father had been away from work for some time and he was looking for a job. I was alone and I knew I would have to speak to my son soon. I realized that I hadn't made any notes, not one, about what the doctors had told me, and was lost in the details.

Samer called me, still confused. Samer had many questions and I couldn't answer them all. I could hear his frustration and fear. But I was unsure what all this information meant. What would we do? I felt that we would have to trust a doctor and place our faith in them, no matter what. I knew that despite my questions, there was a part in me that had already decided this.

Throughout the ordeal, I felt immense pressure to follow all instructions. It was exhausting to absorb so much information. I was frequently left with questions, and sometimes misunderstandings. Because I was given medical opinions as facts and had no other options, I didn't know what questions to ask. It was often difficult for me to recall conversations from just a few hours ago or who was there then!

I tried to remember to bring a notebook to jot down the information, but it was difficult. I found it helpful to have someone with me so that we could continue the conversation.

I learned to not be afraid to ask the doctor for a repeat of my question. They are experts, but not "authority." I realized they were there to help me make the best decisions for my child.

The first day I went to work, I was totally unprepared. I had no paper, no pen. I didn't know what I would hear and was so shocked that I couldn't help Samer with his questions.

Samer called his family in Lebanon immediately after he hung up. Everyone was calling their doctors to find out what Ewing's Sarcoma was. All their search results and advice would soon be flooding in fast and furious. Although I was aware they wanted to help, it only made me more anxious.

The word quickly spread among our friends, family, and acquaintances. People looked around the globe to see what Yousef had. The opinions began to circulate: Go to Italy, Beirut, USA, and go straight to Sweden.

I managed to make it down the corridor to Yousef's room. He was still lying on his back. I tried to stop myself from crying, so he wouldn't be scared.

"I'm going downstairs for the coffee shop. "Would you like some?" I asked.

"No," he said.

I walked out of that room in a trance with the same thought replaying in my head: Your son has cancer.

I went to the coffee shop and was totally numb. Salina, my daughter, called me. Although she doesn't usually pick up the phone at work, she did this time.

"The doctors came and spoke to me. They said that Yousef had cancer. It's Ewing's Sarcoma, they think," I said to them. Salina later told me how strange my voice sounded.

I heard her scream on the other end of my phone. My face began to well up with hot tears. As a robot, my eyes widened as I moved in line for a latte. The people there thought I was insane. Maybe they're used to it?

Salina said we would speak to Yousef together. UAE family is first. So when she informed her employer about the incident, they allowed her to leave work and come be with us.

Because Yousef was my mother, I was close to the situation, so emotionally involved that Salina took control of the situation when I needed it. Yousef had an extra mother in Salina. She has been caring for her brothers and sisters since she was a small child. Salina stated that she knew right away that her role was to support Yousef and that she would support me. Without her, I wouldn't be able to do it.

"What should I say to him?" How do I tell my son he has cancer? "How do you tell your child that you have cancer?" she asked. I had so many questions.

She said, "Let's call Lara in the UK." Lara was also her clinical supervisor. "Let's find out what she recommends." "What about Nathalie or Laith?" I ask.

Salina replied, "Don't worry Mamma, we'll tell them.".

After a long time, I finally settled down at the cafeteria's entrance. Tears were streaming. I didn't mind that people were passing me by, even though they were all around me. When I got back upstairs to Yousef's room, it was already past midnight.

had gotten myself together.

Yousef asked, "Where have you been for so long Mamma?".

"Oh, it took some while to get the coffee," I replied.

My darling son, he was playing in his bed. My mind was racing with thoughts. What if he dies? I wondered. What could I do to help him? What can I do to tell him the terrible news?

Now, I am reminded of how far I had been away from him and wonder what he was thinking. Is it a bad thing that I am a mother? It wasn't an intentional decision to leave, but I was trying my best to keep one foot in front the other. It wasn't perfect but it was enough.

Later that afternoon, Yousef had an MRI scheduled. This was a huge deal for him.

He said "No!" "I'm not going in there!"

I wish someone had explained to him why he needed an MRI and how it would work. No one explained it to him, and I didn’t have enough information to explain it to him. It was difficult for a nine year old boy to deal with the shock of breaking his leg twice and being admitted to the hospital.

The machine's noises terrified him during the test. He found every test and procedure difficult after this traumatic experience. It was difficult to let go of the fear that was already instilled in him. He would eventually have to undergo anesthesia for the majority of his scans. It would have been a great help to him to be able to relax for his first MRI. It taught me a lot about how to talk with my son and how to help him manage his anxiety and fear as we went.

My anxiety was also a constant struggle. I had very little time to process my emotions which would have been helpful for him. Even though I was unsure of what to say, I couldn't wait for my children and friends to speak to me. I hoped that someone would be able to help me find the right person or give me the right advice. Samer would soon be back, and we would talk about the best options for Yousef.

Accepting What Is

It doesn't matter how you hear it, whether you thought something was wrong, if you were alone or with someone, the shock of hearing the diagnosis will surprise you. Your life will be forever changed by this diagnosis.

What's the best thing you can do right now?

Your partner/spouse may have different communication styles, questions and reactions than you.

What's the gift between you in all these differences?

Well-intentioned people will give you a lot of information.

What if they feel better because of all the research they do? It doesn't have to be about you. Let that be?

Your child may have difficulty with negative news, tests and procedures, just like Yousef. A friend of mine tells her 7 year old son that he will be having a blood test. He panics. He then goes back to his bedroom and comes down, fully prepared to take the test.

Imagine if your child could tell what is best for you. What if you didn't hesitate to ask your child and trusted their deep wisdom?

My Notes

CHAPTER TWO

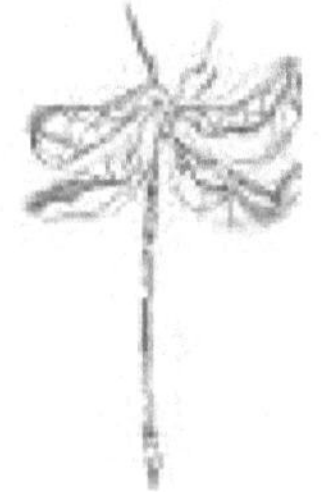

Will I Die?

"When we face death, face it really, we realize that love is all that matters."

– Marty Rubin

L Salina and me sat down that afternoon with Yousef. He was aware that he had more to his broken bone.

"We need to tell you something important. Salina stated, "We heard back about your tests." She stopped and listened to Yousef's reaction.

She pointed at his leg. They believe it's cancerous in your bone. It broke again three weeks ago.

Salina waited while Yousef was being taken care of. She was calm and reassuring. She was careful to keep every sentence brief. She explained that she was now in her professional mode and used "therapeutic pauses" just like she did with her young clients.

Salina assured him that no one would be shocked to hear such news. She kept her pace so that she didn't overwhelm him by details, she also mentioned other family members who had been diagnosed with cancer.

"You all know Uncle Omar had cancer. He received special treatment and was able to recover. It was the same for Auntie Jill, and Auntie Liselotte.

We did not include people who had lost their battle with cancer. Salina informed Yousef that a biopsy would be required by doctors.

"The doctors take a small piece of bone for the lab to examine." They'll then determine what kind of cancer you have, and the best treatment.

Salina knew that he would be afraid to hear this. Yousef worried all the time about how it would hurt. If it was an injection, then we would have to tell him that it could hurt. We could also tell him that he would have a quick and painless x-ray if he had been scheduled. He wanted to know about the biopsy.

"You'll fall asleep. It won't be there," Salina stated.

He was actually in severe pain after the biopsy.

We told Yousef we would do all we could to help him, that our friends and family would do the same, as well as doctors and nurses. Yousef stared at us. I thought of what I could do for him to make it more easy. Salina asked him questions.

Yousef asked, "Will you die?" Children can be so blunt!

"God will provide a treatment." She said that everyone is looking for the best treatment to help you get well. "We are also looking to see if you would prefer to travel to another country." Yousef stated.

"OK. Salina stated, "OK.

It was obvious that there was tension in my body and my face. Salina reprimanded me and reminded me that Yousef can pick up on my emotions.

She said that children are more intuitive than they give credit for. He can sense your stress and see your worry. You might be adding more anxiety to his feelings if you don't have the information processed before you speak to him.

Since then, I have been super aware of this. Every chance I had, I would take a moment to look around and breathe. I let myself be aware of the world around me and made it a habit to look for small things to appreciate. Focusing on one beautiful color or scene helped me to stay focused and in the present. This allowed me to remind myself that I have enough time to express my thoughts slowly and in the right manner.

Through the entire process, I was able to see when Yousef had sufficient information. He would curl in on himself, like a snail or a role-poly. It was evident in his eyes when he shut down. He might nod at us, as though he were listening. But his eyes could wander or he might cry. These signs became a sign that we stopped talking and we began to be more sensitive. He could always ask for explanations later, if he so desired.

In the beginning, I felt so much pressure. I needed to gather information. I needed to make quick decisions. I was limited in time to ask the doctors all my questions. I was worried that I might forget something, but it turned out that I had forgotten. Some doctors were patient and took their time. Some doctors made us feel more anxious because they were not very patient or had a poor bedside manner. We were able to overlook arrogance and impatience with some of them because of their confidence, experience, and skill.

I was trying to figure out what Yousef should know and what I needed. Salina was a great help to me as I tried to figure out how I could tell Yousef.

I was going through my own trauma over my child's illness. It can be overwhelming for parents. Salina could tell when I was feeling flustered or in shock. Although she advised me to first process the information myself, I found it difficult to not react emotionally when things were coming at me so quickly.

"How can I comfort him while simultaneously exposing him to these frightening things?" I asked.

Salina stated, "Reassure him!" Even if it's all that you can do. Tell him that you will be there for him, and that you won't be alone. That's enough.

We all believed that it was best to be honest with Yousef. Even though it was hard, we always told Yousef the truth. It is not common for every family to choose this path. When Yousef asked us if we knew when he would die, for example, we said that we didn't.

"Yousef! It's not just kids with cancer," I said. "No one knows when their time is coming," I said.

Yousef was nine years old. We might have done something differently with a younger child, but we decided to take it slow and watch his reactions so that we could tell him the truth. Salina advised us to trust our gut instincts. We gave him something to do if he reached his limit. A toy, TV show, or game. We wouldn't place more pressure on him if it had been a difficult day of treatment or testing. We would let him be.

We let him speak the truth whenever possible. Sometimes he had to know certain things right away. We didn't want him to be surprised with tests or procedures. Without Yousef saying it, we learned to be sensitive to signs that indicated "I'm done!" I would say, "Maybe you don't feel like talking about this now, that's OK, we can do later" or "You can tell when I should stop."

Salina reminded us that when he seemed worried about something, it was OK to ask him, "I wonder what you are worried about?" It was often hard to see his worry on my face.

Yousef switched between asking questions and shutting down. Salina explained to me that "I wonder ..."" is a great sentence starter, and "I don't understand" is also a perfectly acceptable (and honest) sentence. It turned out that there was so much more I didn't know. It was a relief for Yousef and me to allow that to be.

How to Talk to Your Child.

Let them be the ones to follow.

Answer only what they ask. If they don't want more details, don't give them any.

Be honest if you don't have the answer. Let's talk to the doctor.

Take some time for yourself if you feel anxious. This will help you to be calm and relaxed when you speak. You can say, “I want to talk with you about that.” Please give me a hug and allow me to take a few minutes so that I can respond in the best possible way.

If there is news that the child doesn't like, let them know. "Tell him when you're done."

"You can always ask questions. We can always ask the nurse or doctor if I don't understand.

"You can always reach me later."

"I wonder what you feel?"

"I wonder what you would like to know?"

"What would make it easier for you to feel better right now?"

It doesn't matter how often you want to speak, it's okay."

"There are no subjects that are off limits, even scary topics."

"It's okay if you don’t want to talk about the subject."

"It's okay if you don’t want the details."

"Tell me when I've had enough."

“It’s OK to cry.”

"What are you doing right now to feel better?"

My Notes

CHAPTER THREE

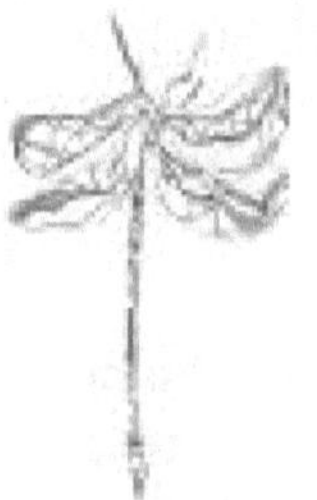

Dr. Who?

"The strength you feel tomorrow is what you feel today." There is always room for growth in every challenge.

—Unknown

My first instinct was to support Yousef by being positive, but it may have been a bit too much! Yousef was admitted to the hospital that night right after his (unconfirmed!) diagnosis. Salina was asked to contact our family and friends to tell them that Yousef could be visited. I asked them to bring smiles and happiness. I asked them to not show fear or worry, but to be positive and support Yousef.

We were surrounded by our family and friends that night. We brought food to his room and held a party. It was a very happy evening for Yousef, with so much attention and so many toys and presents. That is exactly what I wanted. Now, I believe he was overindulged by all the gifts and attention. Maybe he was also confused from having a party after hearing the bad news. He didn't know what was coming. It made me wonder if I was doing the right thing by pumping him up and then having him crash to Earth with what followed. He was not prepared. But how can I prepare a nine-year-old to face cancer treatment in another country and leave his family? How would I get him to understand it all? Now I look back and see how clueless we were all.

That night, I finally fell asleep at home. When something so unexpected happens, it is normal to feel in a trance. You can't function properly, you can't sleep and eat well. You do what you need to do, which is to go to the hospital. Order food. Take care of the little things.

There are also big decisions that need to be made. To find the best possible treatment, we were compiling medical reports and sending them to doctors abroad. We didn't know where to go or what country. Many people offered their help and advice, but we didn't know which hospital would be best for Yousef. Although it was overwhelming, Samer and myself were able to decide what was best for Yousef. Both of us prefer natural healing methods, but when I heard how critical Yousef was, I trusted the doctors.

Nathalie, my younger daughter, was shocked that I even considered chemo. But Salina assured her, "Do what's best to Yousef."

Jill, who is Salina's mother in law and has been a survivor of cancer herself, was my friend. She knew a lot of people in Dubai and other places, and she had also been treated in Germany for cancer. I rely on her strength a lot so I asked her for help. Jill knew of an Abu Dhabi contact who can expedite medical treatment for people who need it. He immediately began to locate doctors for Yousef. We would be paying for the treatment ourselves, so he knew that we needed to keep costs low.

Because we were not Dubai residents, our situation was unusual. We would have been citizens if the government, or a wealthy patron, had paid for our medical care. It wouldn't be uncommon to find wealth in the country, especially if there is a child involved. Yousef, on the other hand could have been treated anywhere in Europe if he were a resident of the European Union. He was not covered because he was a non-resident.

Although I tried to keep the financial side in perspective, it was still something that I thought about as We searched for the best treatment for Yousef's rare form of cancer. We wanted the best for him but did not have enough money to pay for it. Samer was out of work for a while, and our savings wouldn't cover the thousands of euros it would take to pay for his medical care.

Yes, we would have to raise a lot of money. But I decided that I would trust that it would come from somewhere. I needed to believe that the right care would be provided.

Everything I found online was overwhelming. Add to that the sheer number of people searching on the internet! Although the internet is amazing, I would not go there immediately to find information, even though it seems like everyone's first instinct.

It's probably overwhelming when your brain has already been overloaded with information from doctors. Although I am aware that I should only go to trusted sites such as cancer centers and hospitals, the stories of other parents still caught my eye and I decided to not visit them.

Although I wasn't a huge Facebook user, it was a vital tool for many. Facebook is another platform where friends can share the worst stories, cases, and other things that they have heard. It's okay to tell them to stop. I didn't want to tell anyone, but only my "likes" and close friends. Thank you!" Without that, I was at risk of wondering "what happens if all those horrible things happen to my child!"!

One friend of mine asked me to be her contact person. Each day, they would talk and then the friend would post to Facebook. She never replied to any of the comments. Nearly all of the comments were supportive. Only if something was offered of helpful help did she break the rules and tell us.

We need to be in control of our social media use and not allow posts, emails, or texts to overwhelm us. I realized that I didn't need to answer every email or tell everyone everything. I chose to deal with it anyway and not worry about offending anyone!

I wanted to create a blog so that I could keep up with all developments. It would be beneficial for me and let my loved ones know about what was going on. But I was not aware of how much it would involve and what could happen. Although I quickly gave up on the idea, I did take a lot pictures and took notes with my phone so that I could later remember what I had written. I have been able to reconstruct the story using pictures.

We were told by the doctors that Yousef should have a biopsy immediately to determine what type of cancer it was, as well as whether or not it had spread and at what stage. We would have to make a decision right away, as there was no time for us to wait. It was extremely stressful. It was difficult to keep up speed. But now that I look back, I can see the line you cross when it comes to cancer treatment. There is no turning back. It was like we were on a treadmill, and couldn't get off.

We knew we couldn't remain in Dubai because there weren't enough cancer services available for children. I considered returning to Sweden but didn't know how. Throughout this period, people kept calling and offering advice. Jill was trustworthy and I followed her advice instinctively. Jill called me to inform me that a doctor was available to us. I felt a tremendous weight loss and didn't hesitate to follow her advice. I felt hopeful that Yousef would soon be treated. A doctor who is actually knowledgeable about children's cancer would be willing to accept my son as a patient. Even now, months later, I still feel the same chills. It was because that "yes" meant there was hope.

Problem was that I was not processing all the information correctly. After Jill mentioned Heidelberg to me, I began researching and realized that Heidelberg University Hospital was where I would be going to see Dr. Ho. It was not true! Jill's contact in Germany had located a government hospital in Karlsruhe where Dr. Schmittenbecher would be willing to see Yousef immediately. We were as anxious to find answers and begin some type of treatment as possible, but we couldn't help but put him off so that we could arrange travel and take good care of things at home. He was willing to meet us on Monday.

I suppose I thought Dr. Schmittenbecher was an associate with Dr. Ho. Karlsruhe was not in my area of expertise. It's funny to see how ignorant Samer and me were. Who wants to get on a plane and not know where they are going? If you don't know where you are going, how can you read the departures board? Even after the plane landed, we didn't know what to do. We were then met by a stranger, who drove us miles to Karlsruhe in the middle of the night. I had already told everyone about the great doctor and hospital in Heidelberg at home.

"It's world-class treatment, the best and the most prestigious!" I declared, wanting to give Yousef hope and faith.

"You're going into this amazing hospital!" This is a very lucky boy because not everyone gets to see this amazing doctor!

I sent a text to Suzie who had called me when Yousef broke a leg. It said, "Yesterday," and that the best doctor for Yousef's situation agreed to treat him. We will be traveling on Sunday, as he is currently in Germany. I asked everyone to be calm and happy. All I ask is for Yousef to feel secure, safe and happy. It's not a lot for him as a small boy. He is brave and takes a lot of pain.

Samer and Yousef were shocked at how busy I was. They didn't have time to see many people. I played it up and told them how difficult it was to get into the specialist's office. We weren't going see this doctor!

We were still in Dubai and we felt pressured to rush to Germany to get the biopsy. I was curious about how I would get my son there and what he would experience to be cured.

We didn't know much beyond what doctors already said: They suspected Yousef to have Ewing's Sarcoma. This is a malignant, small-sized, round, and blue-cell tumor. It is a rare bone and soft tissue disease. It is most common in the pelvis and femurs. We all know that Ewing's Sarcoma is Googleable. You can find so much information online, which is great. But you end up finding the most horrific cases and horror stories. Every individual is different and each case is unique. Nevertheless, the biopsy was not a guarantee. We were forced to wait and nothing was certain. There was no reason to be upset about what we had read online.

To keep my mental and physical strength, I chose to remain focused, take each day as it came, and do my best to make the most of it. Many people called me to reach out to me. I was grateful even though I could not answer every question or answer all of their questions. It was exhausting to try and repeat the same thing over and over again.

I wrote to Suzie,

God knows best. Whatever I get, I am so grateful. Please keep Yousef in my prayers, even if I can't speak to you. Once I have more information and we reach the destination, I will keep you informed."

Despite my resolves, I was anxious the night before we left Germany with my friends. I believed we had a doctor and an itinerary, so I focused on packing. But the pressure was unbelievable in my head.

My husband was unemployed. He had been searching for work for a while. Our apartment was rented and we had to pay the rent one year in advance. I felt panic and worried that my home might be lost. I felt overwhelmed. I needed my home, my belongings, and my place. At least we knew that we could return home at the end the day at the Dubai hospital. However, there would not be a "home" once we had left the country and moved to Germany. These were all the thoughts that were running through my mind. When I went to Germany, I was unsure if we would ever return. There would be no income, no certainty. Samer would later return to the apartment and live there, but I didn't.

That night I was surrounded by friends, and felt completely overwhelmed as I stood in my bedroom.

Jill said to me that "don't worry" and "Your home will be here."

They all stated, "We promise that your home will be there, and you'll come back,".

They were so convincing to me. Dubai was safe and familiar. I didn't know what was ahead, where we would go, how it would turn out, and, most importantly, who our child would be.

It seems absurd now that I think back. I was trying to protect my belongings - but they are only things. It was my shock and confusion, and it shows how different I am now.

CONTAINER VISUALIZATION

Before you read on, I ask you to take a moment to reflect. You can use this visualization right now to take control of your emotions and thoughts. It is used by therapists to "contain overwhelming feelings.".

Do not worry if visualization isn't your forte. You'll see the results if you do your best. It will become second nature. You'll eventually be able instantly to feel your emotional "breathing space"

Take your time and go slowly through each step. You might ask someone who you trust to read the steps for you. This is a great way to show your child that you care.

Take at least three deep...slow... breathes.

- Allow all your emotions to rise to the surface.
- Imagine putting them all together, with all your emotions and all your
- thoughts.

Imagine all those emotions being placed in a "container."

It can be any type of gift box or cardboard box you want, as well as a tin.

- Watch yourself pour all your feelings in and seal the box. Use tape, ribbon, glue, whatever you like. Seal it up tight so that all the emotions are safely locked up in the box. <u>Take your time.</u>
- Now, see yourself put the box on a shelf in a closet.
- Close the closet door, and lock it. Move away from the door.
-

You can see the door and feel the emotions outside you. They are locked in a box in the locked closet. They are gone for now.

- They are always there if you want to go get them. Maybe you won't.
- Feel the lightness and freedom. Relax and feel at ease. Breathe.

My Notes

CHAPTER FOUR

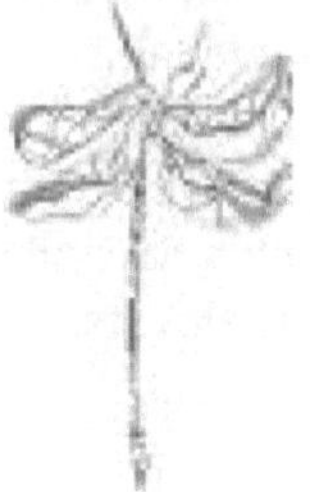

What is the best way to bring happiness?

"Difficult roads often lead you to beautiful destinations."

– Zig Ziglar

Looking back, I should have listened to the first doctor who advised me to "go your country." We should have flown directly to Sweden to get it checked out and then continued our journey. A young boy wouldn't be turned down by them. But I wasn't aware of the possible consequences. We decided to take another route.

Everything was moving at a rapid pace. We left the hospital on Friday night, February 27, to get ready for our trip to Germany. Salina and Jill had purchased Yousef an electric wheelchair so that he could travel on the plane. Jill had done all the paperwork, made phone calls to Germany and made arrangements for hotel rooms and contacts. It was amazing to see how many people would help in such a situation. To make it easier for Yousef, a close friend gave us business class tickets. Because his leg was so severe, he couldn't fit in an ordinary airline seat. We were also helped by generous donations.

We were happy for Yousef the two days before we left for Germany. People were coming over and he was having an ongoing party. Samer and me were both overwhelmed and still in shock. We planned to take our child abroad and we didn't know what to expect. Although I was fluent in German, I had not studied it. We didn't know the details of the treatment protocol, What Yousef would go through, or how long it would take. It was difficult enough to be diagnosed with cancer. It was hard to imagine leaving our country and home.

Yousef was in terrible pain the morning we left. I tried to give him painkillers, but they took quite a while to work. I sat down beside him and sang a lullaby that I used to sing to him as a baby. To help him relax, he asked me to tell the Trouble Tree story.

Lynn, the school nurse, was available to answer my call at 8:00 AM. She asked if Yousef would like to pass before he went to the airport to say goodbye to his friends. She checked with the principal and was granted permission.

Laith, my boy, and Lou, our long-time housekeeper and nanny, rang the doorbell. They had been with me since Salina was three years old. We shared some Swedish Kanelbullar (cinnamon rolls), together. Freshly baked goods make me happy and feel homey. They weren't made from scratch. I purchased them frozen at IKEA so that everyone would think I was up at dawn baking!

We arrived at Safa School at 9.45 am. The school was packed with children who came to the front to sign Yousef's cast. Max gave Yousef an lollipop because it was Max's birthday. He was turning nine. Rayan also told me that it was her mother's birthday. Even amid all the chaos, there was still something to celebrate: family, friends, and birthdays. After taking pictures, we said goodbye to everyone and then got back in the car and headed for the airport.

Yousef was very sad but grateful to have all his friends' names on the cast.

He was not interested in speaking during the drive and asked me to keep quiet. I felt his pain in the pit of my stomach. I thought, "What will it take to bring me happiness?"?

Jill and Salina were following us. At the airport, Samer, Laith and Lou waited for us. Nathalie was not with us, as she was at University in London. However, she would be the first to arrive in Germany. She might feel bad for being so far from home, I was worried.

We arrived at the airport and were able to check in quickly. Laith helped Yousef in the wheelchair to get to the gate. Then it was time for us to say goodbye. It was a long time until we meet again, I thought. It was hard to hold back the tears. It was overwhelming to feel so many emotions about the departure. Although they were brave, I feel very connected to my children and could feel their sadness when I watched their little brother and me depart for another country. They didn't know what was coming, but they knew that I would not be able care for them for long. I could not hug them, comfort them or make them feel safe. Salina, my eldest daughter, told me to not worry and to take care Of Yousef.

She said, "We'll be fine." "Don't worry about me."

I reminded myself that crying wouldn't make things better, not for me nor them. I reminded my self that all my thoughts, emotions, and feelings are in my head. While I couldn't choose the events around me, I could choose how I react to them. I decided that it was best for us all to concentrate on the NOW. It is hard to imagine myself saying goodbye, and I feel many emotions. Although I'm not without emotion, I decided to control my emotions to take better care all of us. It is their mother's job to protect and keep them safe, even though they have grown up. But I remembered that Lou, our long-time nanny, who was a family member, would still be there. Jill, her mother-in-law and our friend, was Salina's friend. I knew that my children had support. This wasn't the end of my life. I understood that caring for my youngest son, who was fighting for his life, was my greatest mission. It was now time to take care of him.

We all wanted to be together on that flight so I prayed and pondered what it would take to upgrade Samer to business class so he could join Yousef, me and Yousef. We parted ways with our families and went to the lounge to see if my husband would be able to join us. Samer was denied access to the lounge while Yousef and me had business class seats.

I was told "OK, but only this once.".

It is amazing to me how many people feel the need to show you how important they are, all just to get you into a lounge. It doesn't matter that the child in the wheelchair in front is going to be treated for cancer and wants to sit with his parents.

All of us got into our seats and settled in. Yousef was tired and fell asleep. After a short nap, Yousef woke up and asked for food. I gave him pasta with tomato sauce, and unhealthy doughnuts and cookies.

After some time, he wanted to use the bathroom, and luckily, it was wheelchair-accessible, unlike many other places. Dubai is still not accessible but it is improving.

When it was time to board the plane I kept asking myself, "What would it take for Samer get upgraded to business-class?" It did shake me a bit when he didn't. I kept asking questions and tried to remain in that state. I thought, "What other possibilities might this journey offer?"

It was a challenge to get Yousef aboard, but it was possible. He felt safe and settled in. He had been wondering about this since we told him we were going to be flying abroad. But it turned out well.

We ordered our food. He enjoyed his soup and felt relaxed as he ate it. We flew smoothly and were met by Jill, a young man who helped us get through customs and immigration in Germany. After we had slept through the night, he drove us to our hotel. It was still my belief that we were heading to Heidelberg. By the time We got into the car, Yousef was exhausted. We drove for more than two hours to Karlsruhe which is south Frankfurt. The hospital was only 30 minutes from our hotel, which we didn't know when we stopped at the hotel. We were told by our driver that a different man would pick us up the next morning and take us to the Klinikum Karlsruhe for Children. I was eager to meet the Heidelberg doctor that I had researched so much for my husband and son.

Jill managed to book us in Erbprinz, a small hotel in Ettlingen. This was a bright spot. We were delighted to discover a small, family-run hotel that would be our comfort for the next three month. I went to bed confident that we would be in good hands once we reached the hospital and that we would hopefully have an idea of the situation with Yousef by morning.

www.erbprinz.de

When I look back at that trip, I realize how fortunate I am to have been Yousef's mother. He wasn't complaining, despite being so tired and in pain. Perhaps he didn't have the words to express his feelings. It's possible that Yousef understood one thing, but not another. He was a child after all.

HOW TO MAKE DECISIONS

1. You may feel shock for a few days or even weeks. It is possible that you are not getting the oxygen you need to function and think clearly. How might a deep, slow breath help you think clearly and function well right now?
2. It's possible to feel like what you hear is completely unbelievable. It was difficult for me to grasp at first. I still feel emotional thinking about that moment and may continue to do so.**Which of these would you like to understand better?**

3. It is tempting to rush, take a decision, answer questions, and choose a doctor or procedure. Do not make any decisions at this moment. Breathe. As I did, you could ask: "What would your child do, doctor?" Another good question is: "Thanks." What time do you need me to make my decision?
4. Who do you want to support you if you feel helpless or alone? Even if that person isn't available, there are others who can help you. You can even get support from me through these words.

5. All feelings are valid. It doesn't matter what you feel. Trust me. How do you feel?
6. **<u>What can your emotions do to help you understand the feelings of your child?</u>**
7. All of your needs can be met. What (or who) can you ask to get what you need?
8. **<u>What more do you need? Tell them if you feel the need to cry without having someone interrupt or tell you that it won't be okay. You are allowed to ask for someone to hug and comfort you. You are allowed to share your feelings with someone.</u>**
9. Yes, it is urgent to take action and get your child in treatment. You usually have one day. Ask questions, talk to someone. No matter how much advice or information you receive from others in your life, it won't be enough. You will never get the perfect answer and will have to make decisions for your child. How do you know what you know?
10. You can make a change, ask for a second opinion or request other options. Or, you can have the doctors speak slowly to help you think clearly and feel calm. You might be surprised at what you can learn from another perspective. What could you learn from another person's perspective?
11. It is important to write it down. Note down what your doctors say. You can start right now on the next page. Write down questions. Write down your thoughts and fears. After you have finished writing, you can take the extra page and rip it out. You might decide to take the list with you and rip it out. You might decide to rip the page out and throw it away, because you believe what you wrote is too horrible for anyone else. You can do it. It's okay. How might that be beneficial?
12. **What's useful about how you feel? As long as you feel it, you can feel whatever you want. It is a journey. It is possible to take each step one at a time. It will be unfamiliar for a while. It's okay to feel a little lost in your surroundings and yourself. It's normal to feel lost.**
13. **Imagine what you could do if YOU took care of yourself. Take care of your child as well as yourself. Ask for help caring for your child. Get help for yourself. Even the smallest things.**

CHAPTER FIVE

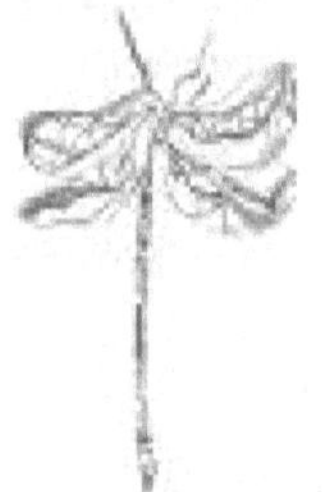

Now We Know What's Next

"Every day is not good, but there are good things in every day."

— Alyce Morse Earl

The next morning, Monday 2nd of March, I woke up hoping that answers would be within hours. In daylight, I could see the warm touches of Erbprinz, such as the small bouquets full of flowers.

The hotel has been given an extra color.

The spa is a lovely addition to the hotel. When we were shown around the place, I imagined myself relaxing in the steam room, surrounded by aroma oils, or on the loungers on the terrace. The spa was not what I expected and I soon forgot that it existed. Samer tried it once or twice, but was shocked by the co-ed sauna full of naked men and women. Samer is more conservative than some Germans who love their spa days. Although I was not able to do the same at home, I did use the gym frequently. It helped me keep up my strength and cardio as well as my yoga practice. The bathtub in our bedroom was large enough that I could take a hot bath with mineral salts before getting to sleep. I needed to find ways I could relax and retreat when I could. Now I can remember how much I enjoyed the baths and how my body felt afterwards.

It is crucial to take care of your body. Your child relies on you. If you're tired or undernourished, your child will be unable to do their best. It is easy to be impatient, overworked, and unfocused. You are important to your child, so make sure you take care of your well-being and health. It's not selfish; it is essential.

Our room had a kitchenette, a bathroom with a wheelchair-accessible door and a bathtub. Although I was unable to allow Yousef to take a bath, I would sponge him in the tub to provide him with the benefits of the soothing sea salts.

The cool temperatures in Germany were not something we were used to after the sun of Dubai. However, it wouldn't matter that much over the next weeks and months since we barely left our hotel rooms or the hospital. As time passed, we would continue to explore Ettlingen, but not with Yousef. He would have to wear a leg cast, which made it difficult for him to travel. Also, as he started his chemotherapy treatments, he felt less well.

Ettlingen is an historic and picturesque little town with cobblestone streets and buildings in classical style. It would make a great place to visit in any other circumstance. I hope to return one day.

My first morning I can remember getting up at 5 am and having breakfast with my mom. At 2:00 PM, a taxi picked us up to transport us to the hospital. We arrived at the hospital thirty minutes later. It was a longer trip than I anticipated, but I ignored any doubts.

Wael, a man from Wael, met us when we arrived at Kinder Klinikum. We would be so grateful to him. He could speak Arabic and German, and would serve as our interpreter. He brought us to Dr. Peter Schmittenbecher who was both a professor and a head of surgery. We found out immediately that he does not perform the type of operation Yousef would require. This frustrated me and left me confused. What were we doing then? He stated that they were treating children in the children's oncology unit, but that some children had to go elsewhere for surgery and return later for their chemotherapy. It was a confusing process. It was enough to confuse me! How would you get the answers you seek?

I was eager to meet the doctor that I had heard so much about and whom I had told Yousef with such enthusiasm. I knew he would be able to answer my questions. I was determined to speak with him.

I asked, "Do you work for Dr. Ho?".

“Who?” Dr. Schmittenbecher said.

I replied, "You don’t know Dr. Ho?".

He didn't know who I was talking to. I was stunned and didn't know how to respond. It must have been an associate of Dr. Ho, I thought. Were we in the wrong spot? They had Yousef’s name and they were waiting for us. He didn't even know Dr. Ho! It would have been hilarious if my child's life hadn't been in danger.

Dr. Schmittenbecher was quick to get to work and stated that he would like to see Yousef’s leg. Although he had seen the scans, he wanted to see the cast for himself. Yousef was concerned. When the nurse used a saw to remove the cast, he actually cut his foot's skin! This accident triggered

Yousef's fear. He was becoming anxious about treatments and tests due to this accident and the MRI he had just a week earlier. Yousef would be in a panic at the thought of having the cast removed. A bad experience in Dubai may have caused him to be afraid of needles. They didn't do anything wrong but Yousef did not forget it.

Because he wasn't getting any exercise, I had to inject him with a blood thinner every day during chemotherapy. The first time it happened, I will never forget. Samer was returning home to interview for a job, and there were only Yousef (me) at the hotel. I refused to give him the shot. It took hours of struggle. I was exhausted, shaking and anxious, and became impatient with my little boy. I felt like a horrible mother. It became easier when his father came back to help with the shots. Yousef started to get better at shooting after a while. Each shot and procedure was made into a game for Yousef to win. He also received a "prize". There are many ways to help children accept the frightening aspects of treatment. You can even distract your child by giving him a toy doll to play with during shots. We were later in Sweden and had a wonderful nurse who would encourage him to sing "Staying Alive!" as he received his injections.

The skin texture of Yousef's leg had changed when they opened his cast. It was surprising to me how swelling the leg looked. We were shown the MRI by the doctor, which showed how the tumor was pushing against the surrounding areas. The doctor told us to return the next day and to check in at the hospital. Yousef would be anesthetized for the biopsy.

Samer and me were both really confused and frustrated. It was like everything was up in the air. We had been hoping to see a different doctor in Heidelberg. But now Dr. Schmittenbecher could only perform the biopsy. The operation would require us to travel to another hospital. Did things change or was I wrong from the start? Nathalie, my daughter, was kind enough to talk to me and promise to investigate the situation.

Wael was so kind and offered to take us back to our hotel. Samer and I both thought it would be more convenient to have a room nearer the hospital while driving.

Samer returned to our hotel room after we settled in, and he tried to find us something to eat. However, Yousef and I were not hungry when he returned. I felt like I couldn't talk to anyone. Yousef Skyped Nathalie and then handed me the phone. I ended up speaking to her about the incident, and it was a pleasant experience when she listened. We went to bed and Yousef had an excellent night of sleep considering the circumstances. I would often tell Yousef "The Trouble Tree" to help him fall asleep. It is a wonderful story that can be read to bedtime and it brought comfort to my son. It's here for your convenience.

The Trouble Tree

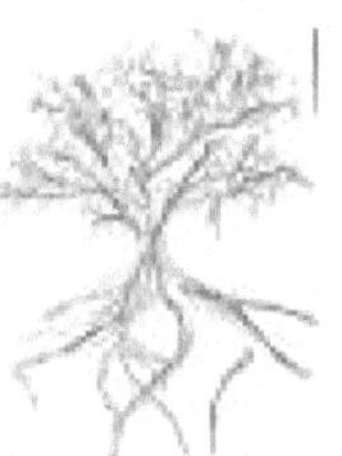

(This is Yousef's and my versions)

This should be read slowly to your child. Pause at the end of each sentence. You might encourage your child to take deep breaths if it is possible for them to do so before you start.

Close your eyes.

Imagine yourself standing in a vast field.

You can see a path, which you will follow.

There is sun shining and a breeze so the grass is moving.

The field is home to beautiful flowers: yellow, blue and some red.

You touch the grass as you walk along the field's path. It feels almost like you are touching it.

Continue walking and you will see a forest at one end of the field. It is so lush and green.

The forest is yours to reach and you can enter it. It's much cooler here. It is almost magical to step in. It feels cooler when you look up at the trees.

The trees move slowly, almost as if they are dancing. You can clearly see the blue sky. You can hear the birds sing. It's amazing how comfortable and relaxed it makes you feel.

You'll be happy to continue on the path. You can see beautiful blueberries as you bend down. They are delicious.

Continue to go deeper into the forest. You suddenly come upon a large wooden gate that looks very old.

You look at me and I will open the gate. You reach for the metal latch at the top of the gate, and you open it.

You can still stand at the gate so that you can ride along with it when it opens. You close the gate behind me as I pass it. We continue walking until we suddenly see a huge tree. It almost seems glowing.

As we walk closer to each other, you stare at me with curious eyes. I explain to you that this tree is special: it's a Trouble Tree. You can forget all your troubles and worries here.

Think about all the problems you've had to deal with today and hang them one by one on the branches.

Let me know when all your worries are gone.

Continue:

Good. Now you can let go of all the things that were bothering your.

After walking a bit, we look back at the tree and turn around.

All your problems are hanging from the tree. They seem distant.

We continue walking and eventually reach the same gate. You open the gate and I enter. The gate is closed behind us.

The path is so pleasant and easy to follow, we continue walking on it. The birds are still singing and the leaves are still rustling in wind. The field we started is now so beautiful, with all its flowers.

You can stay in this peaceful and safe place as long as it is convenient.

After hanging all of his troubles on the tree, Yousef falls asleep almost every night. This story can be told in many ways. You can adapt it in any way you want. Perhaps your child would like to contribute something to make this story more personal.

CHAPTER SIX

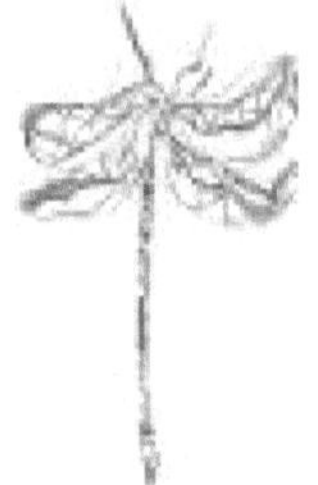

This Is How It Is

We use the thoughts we think to paint our lives.

– Louise Hay

On We woke up on Tuesday, March 3rd and went downstairs to have breakfast. Yousef was full of energy and enjoyed a hot chocolate, an omelet, and sandwich. Although he was nervous about visiting the hospital, there were no issues at check-in. Yousef was given a comfortable, modern room that he felt at ease in. The nurses were extremely kind and accommodating. While Yousef was having tests, Samer and Wael went out to explore the surrounding area.

I asked a nurse what activities were available for the children. I was told by a nurse that there was a playroom next to the hospital and a house out back, which volunteers staffed, so siblings of patients could play.

I thought aloud, "Maybe I could volunteer therefor a few hours" if Yousef would be staying for too long.

I was just looking at the nurse. I didn't know what Yousef was going through. I thought I could do some volunteer work, maintain my fitness, and maybe even do some personal trainer. I didn't know that cancer was going to change my life. It was, however, something that I knew.

I wanted to restore some normalcy in my life and thought I could carry on with my usual activities. Later, the nurse I had spoken to before came back to visit me.

She asked, "Do you know anything about the Eltenhaus?".
Although I assumed she was referring to a home for the elderly, Elten means "parent" in German.

I asked, "Do you think that I should volunteer there?".
She said "No," and added, "That's where you can stay the other parent as only one parent can be in the hospital room at night."

I stared at her, not understanding. I now wonder what she thought about me, a mother who wanted to help her son in his darkest days and to volunteer. However, I think most parents will walk in as I did, unaware of the consequences.

Samer went to the Eltenhaus and returned saying that it was fine. We walked together for a short distance to the Kinder Klinikum. A small room could be used by parents, with a bathroom and a toilet. There was also a shared kitchen and living area. It was a small miracle, exactly what we needed the day before. It doesn't get any better! That's what I thought.

The oncologist Dr. Leipold and Dr. Schmittenbecher visited us at the hospital. Dr. Leipold confirmed that Theresef had a tumor in his leg. He said he would only know the best treatment once the biopsy results returned in 10 days. He could tell us that it would require a lengthy course of chemotherapy. For a year, he would be an outpatient for three to four weeks. He spoke about a similar case that he had three years ago.

He said, "That boy had his cast removed in 6 weeks.".

It was a record time, he said. But Yousef was shocked. Six weeks of walking around in silence? How many weeks without playing football? It turned out that Yousef wasn't as fortunate as the other boy.

Dr. Schmittenbecher said that he would perform the biopsy, but not the surgery. This was a delicate operation that could only be performed by a specialist. He explained it all to Yousef in a charming way. He used the analogy of visiting a village to find out who lives there for the biopsy.

He said, "Before it is possible to know how to treat residents, you must meet them and get to know their personalities." He meant that he didn't know what type of cancer Yousef had until he met them.

Yousef underwent a biopsy on March 4, while under anesthesia. It was hard to describe how it felt to walk away from my child as he went to sleep. I didn't know if he would be awake again. I find it the most difficult thing for parents to do. I watched him get wheeled away and trusted that others would take good care of him. He would eventually go to sleep peacefully, then wake up to look in my eyes.

Yousef felt terrible after the biopsy. He hunched over his leg like he was protecting it. Bone pain is the most severe type. He was fitted with a spinal and could click for morphine whenever needed.

After the biopsy confirmed the diagnosis, Dr. Leipold visited us several days later. We were told that Yousef did not have Ewing's but osteosarcoma. He had to begin chemotherapy immediately. He could now give us more details about the treatment. The first six sessions of chemotherapy would last approximately three months. After that, the tumor would need to be removed. If the leg is clear of cancer, then there will be another round or additional surgery. He stated that the possibility of amputation was possible.

We all stood there in shock, our mouths almost open, and were stunned. We'd had no idea. I tried to find out if there was another way to deal with it.

The doctor stated, "This is how it works.".
"Will your operation be done here?" I asked Dr. Schmittenbecher, who had already explained it to me.

"No, that type of surgery is not performed here. However, you can return to the hospital to continue your chemotherapy for 12 more sessions.

Because they weren't sure how Yousef would respond to the medications, he couldn't give us an estimate of how long it would take. Before they allow you to begin the next round, you must be healthy, have a high blood count, and have no fever or infection. If the child experiences a reaction, infection or has a low platelet count, it can extend treatment for an indefinite amount. If a child has osteosarcoma, they will need to be given strong intravenous drugs to kill the cancer cells. They don't want the cancer to recur. It would be difficult, and Dr. Leipold didn't sugarcoat it. I thought, "Hello! It was not a two-way conversation.

Although I didn't expect it, I was shocked at the medical system. It was not about healing the patient. They only offered chemotherapy. What will it do to him? What will happen to his body? With a jolt I remembered that the doctor had stated that there was no guarantee that his leg would be saved. I had many questions and no doctor was able to answer them.

The pace of things was so rapid that I wanted to know if there were other options. Shouldn't we consider alternatives? This is a child that we are referring to. What are the long-term effects? How will he handle all this? My personal opinion was that chemo would not be performed if I were you. I believe that cures should be found in the ground and I seek out alternatives whenever possible. This was my son. While I wanted to do the right thing for him I felt like I was signing him over to a process that I didn't have good feelings about. It was frightening, unlike anything I've ever experienced before. The doctors did not give me many options. They kept repeating "quickly, rapidly." I couldn't take any chance with my son. When faced with a situation, it is important to decide your course of action and stick with it.

The other aspect of all this was the distance we would be from home. We would be away from home between February and November, if the doctor was correct. It took me months to imagine this. We would never return home, as it turned out. If someone had said that to me, I wouldn't believe it.

Yousef fell apart after the doctor left. He cried, cried, and asked many questions:

"I won't have the ability to walk for a whole year."

"No, that's not what the doctor said," I replied.

"What about school?" PE Swimming? FOOTBALL?" He cried.

I felt terrible for him. It was like his whole life had been taken from him. He was so upset that he crashed and fell asleep. I could not do anything or promise anything to make things better for him. Samer stayed at hospital while I returned to the hotel. Nathalie and I Skyped together, and I didn't fall asleep until 1:00 AM.

"I don't want it!" I kept repeating.

She said she would investigate other options for Yousef and told me to wait rather than to accept the protocol as prescribed by the doctor. It felt like I had no choice and was going to risk my child's health.

Later, I was able to talk to the Eltenhaus coordinator and support person for parents. Claudia asked me about my wishes for alternative solutions.

She said, "You don't have any other choice." "Your son can't go out if you're in the system. It doesn't matter if you are German or not. Another mother was hesitant to sign the paperwork but finally signed it.

Although I knew that chemotherapy was necessary, I decided that I would do my best to make it as natural and safe as possible. For example, I did energy healing on Yousef, asking his body to take the necessary drugs and then dissipate any remaining. I asked God to allow his body to heal and release any harmful substances.

One time, a nurse came into my treatment room during one of my sessions. Although I was unsure of how she would react at first, she eventually said that she could help.

"Wow, this place is full of energy!"

Later, I learned that she was a Reiki practitioner. Whatever anybody thought, if it makes him feel better and I am calm when doing it, it isn't making any worse!

Also, I believe prayers and supplications can have an impact. God is greater than anything we can imagine. God knows exactly what I need, even before I know it. Although I believe in fate, I have the power to make a difference for others and myself. It is possible to choose to be positive and bring hope to any situation. To show my child the positive side of things and to remind him to be thankful for all that is good. Good words and good deeds create positive energy. I believe in God and that it helps me to accept difficult situations. Louise Hay's statement, "I don't fix problems" is something I also believe in. My thinking is what I fix. Problems will then disappear."

I tried to see it all as a positive. But, I kept asking myself the following questions: What will it take to cure Yousef after this whole ordeal? Is it possible for him to feel joy and ease of mind as he heals?

Of course, I still had concerns. There would be many dye and contrast tests and Yousef would need to have anesthesia many times. I was worried to see him undergo anesthesia so many times. He was so stuffed with chemicals that no one knows what the long-term effects will be. Some of these chemicals haven't been around very long. We will have to wait, just like everyone else.

Yousef felt so sick from being injected with medicine that he wouldn't eat certain foods.

"Mamma! Don't give him his favorite foods if he is so sick. Or he will never eat them again. My daughter Nathalie suggested that you spoil them forever.

I am glad I took her advice. Yousef loves sushi, which is his favorite.

Nathalie felt most disconnected from us and was the most detached from all that was happening with her little brother. When We learned that Yousef had died, she was still in London and had just finished her University studies. She had always wanted to go to Dubai immediately. It was just too much time. It was a great honor to be the first to visit Germany with us.

Nathalie and i went shopping together one day to find ways to make Yousef feel better. We also wanted to help him with his treatment. We bought many gifts, both small and large. One jar was filled with different sizes of glass marbles. We wrapped the gifts in small cards and made small notes. Each time Yousef needed medicine, injections or other procedures, we gave them to him. It was an incentive and something he looked forward to. It was a great way to remind Yousef of her support in spirit, even after Nathalie returned from London.

Centering Yourself

Imagine if you could take a few minutes to yourself during tough days. Imagine if you could deliberately put distance between yourself and your thoughts? It might be possible?

Close your eyes, and place your hands on your forehead.

Breathe.

You can feel your face in your hands.

Place your hands on your entire body. Place your hands on your body.

Breathe.

Your feet should be on the ground. Let all your worries and excess energy flow into the ground by letting your feet touch the ground.

You are now fully present. Aware. Be aware:

What can I do today to make it more enjoyable than yesterday?

Breathe.

Alternatives

Alternative treatments, such as diet, herbal, or any other protocol, may have side effects that can affect doctor-prescribed chemotherapy. You might encounter side effects or interactions with chemotherapy drugs.

Are there alternatives to conventional treatments? It seems like people go all-in with the conventional treatment, or they use herbs or supplements to make lifestyle changes. It turns out that many people use milder alternatives or lifestyle modifications in combination with radiation, chemotherapy, surgery or surgery. They might start to meditate or drink more water filtered to flush out the chemicals.

Your doctor should be aware of any changes to your child's lifestyle, diet, supplementary, and other factors as he or she undergoes treatment. Before giving your child any medication, vitamins or other over-the-counter drugs, make sure you consult your healthcare provider.

We did not pursue alternative therapies so I can't speak to their effectiveness. However, I began to use some other treatments after the phase of active treatment.

Lemon Water

Lemon water's purpose is to alkalize the body which can be acidic due to toxins and poor nutrition. Lemon water is a good source for vitamin C and aids in digestion. It also helps to prevent kidney stones. It can be mixed with warm water to flush out the stomach and rehydrate the body. Lemon water is not recommended during chemotherapy because it can make the body very alkaline.

Himalayan Salt

This is believed to be the purest form rock salt. Its iron content is what gives it its pink color. It can be ingested or bathed in, and contains 84 minerals that balance and detoxify. Some people argue that some of these minerals can be radioactive but not enough to cause harm. Himalayan Salt has a high vibrational frequency, which is believed to be healing.

Wheat Grass

Ann Wigmore, a writer in one of the classic books on Wheat Grass usage, writes:

Wheatgrass juice is good for immunity. But, it has other benefits. A number of ingredients in wheatgrass juice have been identified as powerful anti-cancer agents.

One of these is abscisic Acid.

This is a type of plant hormone that prevents seeds from germinating until the environment conditions are right. Wigmore says even small amounts can be fatal to any type of cancer.

Vitamin B17, also known as laetrile, is another powerful contributor to wheatgrass's anticancer properties.

Wigmore writes,

"While the use of laetrile (as a treatment for cancer) is still controversial in the US, the facts are clear: The modern diet contains approximately 400 times more vitamin B17 than that of natives from countries with very low cancer rates.

Wigmore recommends wheatgrass to be used as a tonic, medicine, and an adjunct to your diet. It's natural benefits include a shiny hair and the healing of serious and chronic illnesses like cancer. (See The Wheatgrass Book by Ann Wigmore, Avery Press 1985.

Cannabis Oil

There are many studies that show cannabis oil can cure cancer, diabetes, and fibromyalgia. There is serious research underway and preliminary findings suggest that cannabis oil may have several medicinal properties. Patients tolerate it well and can use it in many ways. For more information, see www.cureourowncancer.org (among other sites) for more information.

My Notes

CHAPTER SEVEN

What Did I Know?

Our lives have many challenges that will help us to believe in ourselves. They're not meant to be a burden.

— Nick Vujici

Y On March 20, Ousef began his treatment. Now that I look back, I see that we didn't really know anything. We didn't know what was coming. I didn't think about what the future would bring. We were simply following the instructions and going. We knew that we couldn't wait. There was no time for waste.

Six treatments were expected, followed by an operation and 12 rounds of chemotherapy. It was discovered that the US, the UK and Northern Europe all use the same protocol.

All of the statistics regarding osteosarcoma were available. We also compared the results from different protocols to see how they compare. It is more common in boys and affects about 3% of children. It has a 70% survival rate. Although I didn't know it at the beginning, I was thankful that Yousef did not have metastasis. After his July operation, they confirmed this. To confirm the bone had not spread, they had to "decalcify" it.

We saw firsthand the many factors that could cause delays in treatment. It was fevers, high white cell counts, low platelets, and infections that Yousef experienced. I found it difficult to comprehend the idea of amputation on his leg, no matter how bad the chemotherapy was. They would be cutting into the bone of his leg! We still didn't know the surgeon who would perform the operation. We weren't aware of all the options available and we were constantly being told by different people which hospital would be best for treating a child with osteosarcoma. This is very rare.

Take one thing at a given time. Chemotherapy.

Yousef was anesthetized to have his port inserted on March 20th. It was placed in his ribs, not his shoulder, as it is more common in other countries. They were shocked to find the port in his ribs when they arrived in Sweden.

We moved to the oncology floor the same day that the port was placed. This is where Yousef started his treatment. He was not able to take a break. The first round of chemotherapy was brutal. They started him with Methotrexate for 24 hour, then followed by Leucovorin for 24 hours. This is a similar compound to Folic acid. Although it is not a chemotherapy drug, it has been used in combination with chemotherapy drugs for years to increase the anti-cancer effect of certain drugs and decrease side effects.

Yousef was fine the first day. But the second day, Yousef began to vomit and had diarrhea. It was horrible - I'd never seen anything similar. He also had to take antibiotics. He couldn't swallow them because he was so nauseated and afraid of vomiting.

Later, we would find out that not all countries handle antibiotics in the same way. We expected our child to swallow them orally even if they couldn't keep it down. To beat an infection, Yousef was only given antibiotics in Sweden if he had a fever.

Although it was difficult to see how sick he was, the nurses were able and compassionate. It was all new to my and I was in shock so the night nurse stayed in our room. She was calm and strong. Although she tried homeopathic remedies to ease the nausea, Nothing could stop Yousef from vomiting.

I was curious if it was normal to have diarrhea and vomit so often.

The nurse stated, "Every child is unique.".

Now I understand that Yousef was very sensitive to the drugs. It was unbelievable to me what chemo did for my son. It was something I had never expected. He received three drugs in the course of his treatment. Two were combined and one was taken on its own. One of the drugs would make him feel more nauseated, while another would have less side effects.

Yousef was also plagued by thrush, or sores on his lips and mouth after the chemo destroyed his natural flora. His mouth was constantly rinsing, his lips were bleedin' and he couldn't eat because of the pain. He rinsed his mouth like mad to stop the sores from returning. Coconut oil was a good option. He used it on his lips and in the mouth. He was so pleased with the results that he was glad to have it.

The hospital switched to tablets after the first, difficult treatment. It was unbelievable to me that they told us they wanted us to "flush" the system at home, which for us was a hotel located 30 minutes away. The flush is done in a hospital in Sweden. Once the chemicals have been reduced to a minimum level, you are not allowed to go home. While we were in Germany Yousef would be released by the hospital and we would go back to our hotel to administer this medicine to him every six hours. I would have to wake him up and ask him to take Leucovorin. I was afraid I would go insane. I still remember the German words I was given to me.

It is crucial to give it to him every 6 hours!

Even Yousef recalls the Germany of that time, "They were very strict there," says he.

Since Samer was back in Dubai for a job interview, I was all by myself with Yousef. I didn't have anyone to turn to, so Yousef was my only support. Because of the things I asked him to do and how frustrated I would become with him, I felt terrible as a mother. Although I wanted to save my son, I felt that I was only adding to his suffering. He was scared to get sick and felt so sick that he couldn't imagine swallowing pills. I was responsible for administering daily injections and antibiotics to him, as well as the "flush" every six hour. It was exhausting. It was exhausting. Yousef was "home" with herbal tea and homeopathic pills to help him manage side effects. It was sage, chamomile, and not very efficient.

Ironically, Samer worked only on and off for the past two years. Then, when his child is sick, Samer gets called to interview in Dubai. Samer hesitated about going, but I encouraged him. He believed it was his responsibility to provide financial support for us. Although it was difficult without him, we did sometimes have disagreements over how we approached issues. So, looking back, it was a good decision that he left. He was also under immense pressure from the high cost of treatment, which made it difficult for him to be productive. Yousef still feels a bit angry about his father's absence. Because Samer isn't allowed to work in Sweden, where Yousef lives now, we don't still live together.

After the second treatment, Samer returned to Germany. Yousef, who woke up the third day after his second treatment, said that he felt "good" and that he was waking up from a three-day nightmare. Samer took over the shooting of Yousef's leg and it was much better for us all. In April, he left again. After that, it was only Yousef, me, and I couldn't leave, even for a moment.

After bloodwork, Yousef was released from the hospital one day later, just a few weeks after his treatment began. To ensure he continued treatment, his blood had to be checked regularly.

He hugged me and said "Mamma." He was firm and quiet. "My hair is coming out of my head when I run my hands through it."

"It's okay, your hair will grow back my darling," I replied. This was a difficult situation for him. But I didn't want it to be a major deal. He was excited to play his Wii U game. Yousef says that I am wrongly stating that it is the Wii U, but that's not true. He reminds me that it was not Laith who gave it. It was the father of a child, a patient, who gave the game to Yousef. It brings back memories of how cloudy my memories can be. I am touched that someone would buy my son this toy for him because he believed it would make him happier.

I prepared mujaddara with cucumber and yogurt salad for Yousef, Samer and Samer that afternoon. Mujaddara is rice mixed with lentils and onions that has been cooked to a soft consistency similar to risotto. It was simple for Yousef. Samer and me talked while I prepared the food and Yousef was in another room.

Samer stated, "I don’t know what I should say to him regarding his hair.".
"I don’t want him to get upset about it," I replied. "He'll only get more upset."

We waited for Salina, who was coming from Dubai, that afternoon. Although she had safely landed, her luggage was missing. She was still waiting at the airport to see if it was on the next flight. I met her at the station, but her luggage hadn't arrived. It was a ridiculous inconvenience considering everything else that we were experiencing. It was wonderful to see my beautiful daughter. Yousef, upon seeing her, was also happy when we arrived at the hotel.

Yousef refused to come down to breakfast the next day. It was probably because of his hair. But maybe he wasn't feeling well enough to go. We all went to the hospital later for his blood test. He pulled at his hair and watched it fall out in horror as he drove. As we waited, he began pulling out more hair, pulling faster and quicker, so that we were all shocked. Salina spoke quietly to him, and told him that he could shave his hair later. Samer was expecting this day. Before returning to Germany, he had shaved his hair to show solidarity with Yousef.

Although Yousef seemed panicked, Yousef believed it wasn't so big YET. Vin Diesel, whom he loved, was already bald. And, anyway, he still had eyebrows and eyelashes. You look different after you lose them, and he was very self-conscious about it.

Salina and me did everyday things like laundry, shopping and walking around town the rest of the day. Her bags were waiting for us when we returned. We took Yousef into the bathroom to shave his head. It was quite shocking, as Yousef refused to go downstairs for breakfast the next day.

We tried to take in the sun from time to time. We went to Ettlingen's lake, unaware that chemotherapy can make the skin extremely sensitive. We should have been more cautious. Yousef stated, "I miss the sun on mine face.".

Sometimes the treatments were very heavy and Yousef became weaker so it was more common to interrupt the routine. Yousef may have high white cell counts, low platelets or fevers. He might be unable to keep up with his treatment schedule due to any of these conditions. He was to receive one treatment and then another followed by two weeks of rest.

I was anxious to get my treatment back on track after he had his first interruption. After a while I realized that it gave Yousef some relief, which I found not so terrible. When he was undergoing chemotherapy, I worried about what it would do to him.

Yousef was restricted in his diet because Germans are strict about food. He couldn't eat any stone fruits or raw vegetables. Only apples, bananas and pears were allowed. He refused to eat any food prepared in the hospital. It was great that I could cook in the Eltenhaus. We were told that Yousef could only eat bland food. This was something we couldn't grasp. I didn't know what to feed him. Later, while we were in Sweden they had a completely different philosophy. It was better for the child eat what he likes as long as it is healthy. Yousef's advice is to let the child eat whatever they like.

It was a blessing that Yousef did not have to use a feeding tube like some other children. Although he did lose some weight, he avoided having to use the tube.

My aunt is extremely knowledgeable about macrobiotic diets. She suggested I do it with Yousef and gave me The Cancer Prevention Diet. The book is packed with information and provides a guide for different types of cancer. The one for bone cancer was the one I used.

Yousef enjoyed the Macrobiotic diet, which is mainly brown rice. It was boiled as porridge and was easy to digest. It is recommended that you start with a few simple preparations: brown rice, miso soup and one sea vegetable. Avoid meat and fish. If the patient craves it, white-meat fish can be enjoyed once every ten to two weeks. You can then gradually increase the variety of natural foods you choose and add new cooking techniques. It is important to move in the right direction. It's about building endurance. We were fortunate to find many organic shops in Germany, so we stockpiled.

We made changes to the macrobiotic diet. Yogurt felt cool in his mouth so I gave it to my son, even though it wasn't macrobiotic. Later on, I was able to add lentils or beans to his diet and he liked them so it was easier to feed him. In Germany, I was more strict with him, and I followed their protocol. However, I was worried when they refused to recommend any raw vegetables or fruits. The Swedish idea that the child could eat what he likes was a great one. Yousef would initially protest at being offered something forbidden, despite the warnings. I had to convince him that it was okay and that it was better for him to eat it.

Chemo had made him resent so many foods that he won't touch anymore. This was his only lasting reminder of those good days.

Terrible Thoughts are Normal

Sometimes, we can have horrible thoughts. These thoughts are normal. These thoughts are more likely when we are stressed or going through difficult times. Sometimes our thoughts might surprise us or embarrass. They might make us feel "bad" about having them. We might be ashamed to even think about them. We aren't necessarily bad people. We are perfectly normal! We are all very normal! Let go of the thought. Breathe in and let it go.

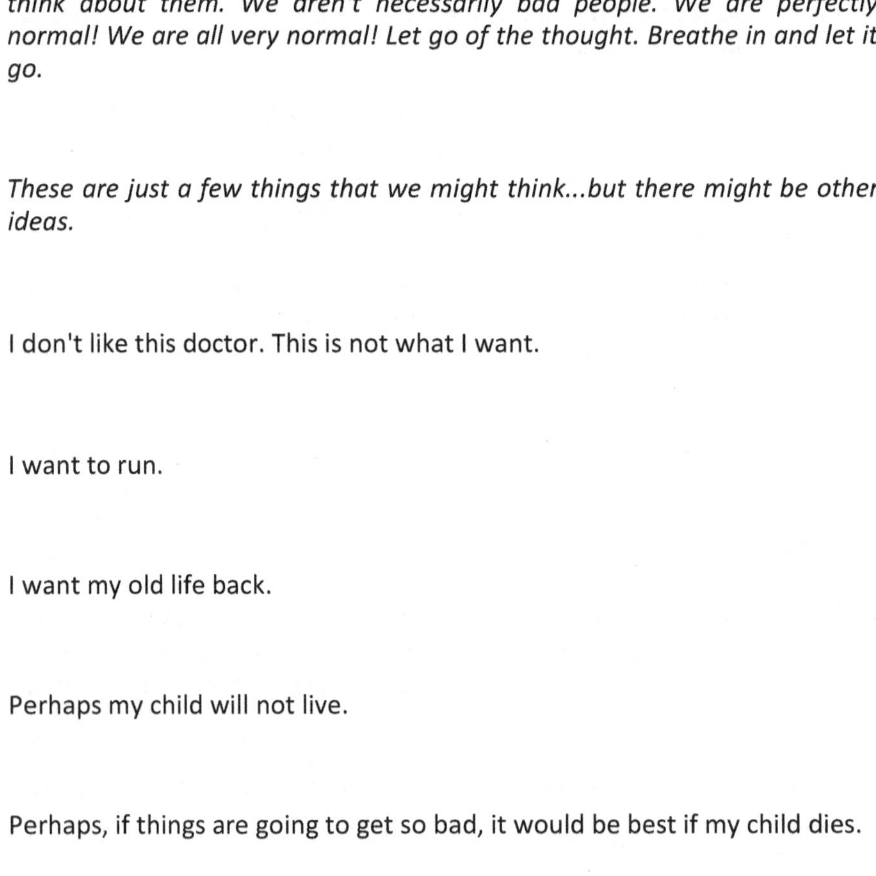

These are just a few things that we might think...but there might be other ideas.

I don't like this doctor. This is not what I want.

I want to run.

I want my old life back.

Perhaps my child will not live.

Perhaps, if things are going to get so bad, it would be best if my child dies.

I cannot stand my wife/husband. I wish they would leave me alone and let me deal with this.

I wish I could just let my wife/husband handle it.

Is there a reason God did this to me?

What are these doctors' secrets?

My useless family is where? They aren't helping me more?

I hate my family.
Once this is over, I will never speak to _________ ever again.

It will never end.

I cannot take anymore.

I cannot be there to watch my child ________.

No one cares.

I feel like I'm neglecting other children.

My children will be left to fend for their own for a while.

I'm a terrible mother/father.

I caused this illness.

My child/husband/mother/other caused this illness.

We wouldn't have all this if we hadn't ___________.

Also, acknowledge your thoughts and feel free to let them go:
Anger.
Shame.
Fear.
Guilt.
Grief.
Doubt.

Please fill in the form below:

Is there anything else? Is your child having terrible thoughts? If your child is open to sharing his or her thoughts, tell him/her that it's okay.

My Notes

CHAPTER EIGHT

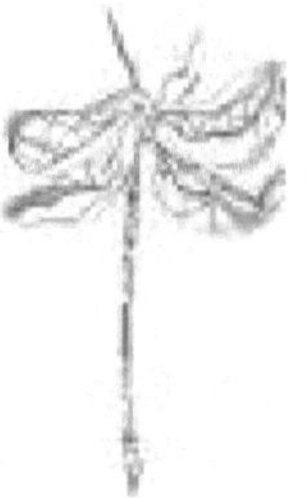

Could It Come Back?

Courage is the most important virtue of all because it's without courage that you can't live up to any other virtue.

— Maya Angelou

O In addition to all the other treatment going on, I was also thinking about the surgery Yousef would have to perform to remove the tumor. I did a lot of research and searched the internet for advice. I also called doctors from all over Europe. Dr. Leipold informed us which European centers are skilled in cancers such as Yousef's. I then narrowed the list to three hospitals: one in the UK where my children were, one in Sweden where I would be (a huge plus), and one in Heidelberg, the place that I believed was the answer to my prayers just a few months ago.

I tried everything to get to the UK. But when we discovered that they would not accept us unless we could afford the surgery, it was impossible to do so. To meet the surgeon, I traveled down the list to Heidelberg. Between chemo treatments, we traveled together until Yousef was able to travel. It's a beautiful city, south of Frankfurt. It was spring and the cherry trees were in full bloom. It was much warmer than Karlsruhe.

I tried to be positive and made a point to notice the beauty in everything around me. I refused to give up and let cancer take over my life. As Yousef was recovering from surgery, I imagined that we would be living in beautiful Heidelberg.

I thought, "OK, I will be here alone, I will live at the hospital, and then we will return to Karlsruhe after the operation.".

We met with a surgeon who drew a diagram showing Yousef's leg. She also described how she would drill into his bone. After examining the bone condition, the surgeon would determine whether an internal or external prosthetic would be best. This would allow Yousef to grow his leg bone. She demonstrated how it would work.

Yousef stated, "I don’t want to put it in!".

According to the doctor, unless she opens up her leg, she would not know if she could put in a prosthetic. Yousef may still lose his leg.

"Oh my God," I cried. "We had no idea!"

Also, I thought "The kid is right here while we talk about cutting off his leg!"

Perhaps we should have spoken up about Yousef to the doctors, but he later told me that he was happy that he was present to hear all of our thoughts. It is not clear what advice I would give another parent. It all depends on the child's maturity and age. This is something that will need to be discussed over and over again throughout the entire process. Some things are possible for the child to hear.

Yousef asked, "Could it return?" He thought back to all the things he had done and was now facing a new challenge. He naturally wondered: If I go through this, can you guarantee that cancer will not come back?

She answered, "Yes," It could return, yes. It could come back, yes. But, it is possible for anyone to get sick at any moment.

I was impressed by her honesty and I personally agreed with her: illness and death can't be denied. But, I do not want to live with that fear and neither did Yousef.

After spinning our heads with all the information, We returned to Karlsruhe to continue our chemo. Yousef felt exhausted for the next two weeks, but he was able to smile on days. To prevent him from experiencing the nausea and vomiting he had experienced previously, they gave Yousef Emend during this round. It did help a little. He still had terrible stomach pains and severe mouth ulcers. Because he couldn't eat, he avoided eating. He was also unable to go to the toilet because he had his leg in a cast. He believed it was better to not eat. Because I could tempt him with them, I allowed him to have things that weren't strictly on the German doctors' diet. If we could, I would avoid a feeding tube.

After the treatment, we went to the hospital for two weeks and Yousef's father returned to Dubai. Samer was not seen again until August, which was quite a while after Yousef had his surgery. It was difficult for Yousef not to be with his father. He didn't understand why he wasn’t there for his surgery.

The hospital where the tumor would have to be removed was still up for me. I reached out to friends, acquaintances, and anyone else in the world who could give me guidance. A friend in Dubai, who is a heart surgeon, connected me with Dr. Cyril Toma from Austria, an oncology specialist who works in Abu Dhabi. I cannot express enough how much Dr. Toma helped me. He suggested we travel to Sweden. He suggested that the London and Heidelberg doctors were highly skilled, but the following-up care was just as important. The recovery process would take many years. Yousef should be monitored for at least 10 years!

Ten years. I was convinced to move to Sweden instead of being alone in Heidelberg for ten years. I wanted the surgery and long-term care to be done in the same location. We should settle down to a routine at a familiar place. We would be able to help Yousef if he had any future problems or complications. That was the end of it. I was going to Sweden and nobody was stopping me. Problem was, nobody was calling me back.

Dr. Toma spoke with an old professor in Sweden who suggested a surgeon, Doctor Otte Brosjo. It was difficult to get in touch with him and it was critical that I did so quickly. I was confused as to why he didn't return my calls. Perhaps he was too busy to perform the surgery. The prosthetic device needed to be made specifically for him. Perhaps he wasn't sure it would be ready in time to meet Yousef. I was so determined at this point that I wanted to jump on a plane and wait in the ER.

In a desperate moment, I called Dr. Toma to plead with him. He wanted to know Dr. Otte’s number. Dr. Otte then sent me an email the next day. Although I didn't ask Dr. Toma what he said to Dr. Otte I am grateful for his reply!

Dr. Otte is a remarkable man. He is passionate about what he does and works from conviction. He sat down and spoke to us with a relaxed and positive attitude when we met him. He assured us that everything would be okay. He made me feel so relaxed. He is the type of doctor who doesn't ask his assistants for help – he does it himself. He is still an educator and a member of the Sarcoma Group of Scandinavia.

The best thing about Yousef's surgery and the follow-up treatment in Sweden was that physiotherapists collaborate with surgeons. This ensures that the surgeons know how to properly train and rehab the patient after the operation. The machine that will insert the prosthetic is designed to gradually lengthen the leg. These two items work together so you need to use the same manufacturer for both the insert and machine. Yousef would also receive physiotherapy to improve his balance, walk and strength.

The prosthetic is precisely placed in the patient's leg by the therapists. It is difficult to train Yousef because his knee is so close to his. Dr. Otte worked closely alongside the therapists in order to determine the best way. It was truly a team effort.

It is important to mention that Dr. Otte never mentioned Yousef losing his leg, unlike the German surgeon. The prosthetic was ordered by him and that was it. After we selected the doctor and hospital, it was time to plan how we would get there and how we would pay.

You worry about your child's ability to take his medication, keep on the treatment schedule and get him to eat. You worry about how your child is handling emotions and how you will take care of yourself as well as the rest of the family. You don't need to worry about how you will pay for the care and surgeries your child requires. I decided to not worry about the money but to trust that it would come. We were prepared to take on debt, and then worry about repaying it later. We were still worried about the cost and the urgency of Yousef's situation, Samer's absence, extended unemployment, and the timing.

We wouldn't have any worries about medical care if we lived in Sweden. However, our situation as non-residents and ex-pats meant that we had to be concerned. The cost of the surgery was estimated at 100,000 Euros. This would cover ten days in hospital. However, it did not include additional costs if Yousef needed to stay longer or required additional hospitalizations due to complications or infections.

Jill had helped us get into the Kinder Klinikum Karlsruhe by arranging support through a friend of a prominent Abu Dhabi man. We were arranged by a close friend to purchase plane tickets to Germany. Others paid for our hotel stay in Ettlingen. All hospital bills in Germany were paid from abroad.

A fee was required to enter Sweden. This made me feel unwelcome even though I was a Swede and that of my child. I had to pay a huge price. I was advised by people to go to Sweden to get emergency care. They wouldn't refuse a child and there is an EU agreement that covers this. I wasn't sure what that would mean and didn't want any chance with Yousef's healthcare.

Samer's uncle paid for our hospital fees. Since Yousef was a Swedish citizen, I knew that once he signed into the country, he would have the same rights to medical care as any other citizen. If you are a Swedish citizen, the Swedish system is fantastic. Both parents are entitled to family leave for a sick child or the birth of a child. However, since I had not lived in Sweden for 25+ years, I was not eligible for any of these benefits.

I would not be able to take sick leave to care of him, or any other non-employment benefits. We were able to get some assistance, which is better than nothing. That is what I am grateful for!

I didn't know how the finances would turn out at the time. I did not know that funds could come from so many people and places. A staggering amount of money was raised through garage sales and fund-raisers sponsored by Yousef and our friends. It was overwhelming to receive support, and I am grateful. I plan to pass it on, at least in part, through this book. Support and generosity can be so encouraging and touching when so much is stressful for a family. It lifted me up when it was hard and gave me hope that everything would turn out well.

My friend had warned me about the Swedish bureaucracy. But it wasn't as bad I expected. They sent me the paperwork and I dealt with everything by phone and mail. Cecilia, my friend from Sweden, called me and took me to Stockholm's Care. She was my guarantor in Sweden.

After deciding that Sweden was the best location for Yousef's rest, we were granted permission to travel and received the funding. We had to figure out how we would get there. I knew that we couldn't fly, no matter what the reason. It would have taken less than two hours but I wasn't sure how Yousef would do on the plane so we decided to drive. It was an amazing adventure that I will never forget. We were on a mission! It was not possible, but it was impossible. I chose to think like Audrey Hepburn who stated, "It's possible!"

Grounding Exercise

This exercise might help you if it feels overwhelming and your head is spinning. You are likely overwhelmed by information, emotions, personalities, demands, and, most importantly, anxiety and fear.

We often get so caught up in our thoughts that we don't see the bigger picture. It's OK. You will feel more grounded and clearer if you allow your energy to return to the earth.

This can be read aloud or given to someone else. Once you are able to do it correctly, you will no longer need to read it. You will have another tool in your arsenal, ready to go whenever you need it.

This is a great meditation to read aloud to your child if you are seeing that he or she is struggling.

* * *

First, if possible, place your feet on the floor and sit straight up in a chair. Once you're comfortable and seated, you can start.

Pay attention to how you breathe. When we are in distress, we often only breathe from the top of our lungs.

Take a moment to notice.

Feel the depth of your breathing.

Once you feel ready, simply tell your body to slow down. Let it slow down.

Let it grow. Do not force it or "intend" to do so.

Allow your breath to sink and allow it to take up more space within your diaphragm.

For a few moments, breathe in the deeper place.

Allow your breath to settle deeper into your belly.

Bring your attention to your feet on the ground. Now, feel the contact between your soles and the sock... the shoe... and finally the ground.

Imagine you are inhaling all the way from your nose, to your lungs, diaphragm and belly, up to your feet, legs, legs and feet.

All of you breathes.

You are all receiving the energy and peace of your breathe.

Imagine your feet are now beginning to root.

The roots reach the floor below.

Roots dig deeply into the soil.

They reach the core of the earth, digging deep into the ground.

Your roots are now in this earth, in this ground you are connected to.

Allow the roots to grow deep and strong.

Feel grounded.

All of the thoughts and feelings that swirl now have roots.

All of them will go right through your feet. All negative emotions, anxiety, and questions.

Let them go from your body into your feet into the earth.

Earth is your anchor, your root, your ground. It does all of this for you and provides support.

The energy flowing from your head, throat, chest, belly and abdomen flows through your feet into the earth.

Feel your feet on the ground. You will feel the roots sinking, anchoring you.

You are solid now.

You are strong.

You have a steady energy.

You are calm.

You can always ground yourself in this way at any moment and feel the power that lies at the root.

A CONVERSATION WITH MARCUS' MUM

Maria, Marcus' mother, is the subject of this interview. She was diagnosed in June 2015 with clear cell renal sarcoma. This conversation was translated from Swedish.

Me: How have your children's experiences with cancer influenced you?

Maria: Maria has always been easy-going. This trait has also influenced my parenting role. When the diagnosis arrived, everything was thrown at us. I felt overwhelmed by the severity of the situation. My realization was that my child cannot have a normal, trouble-free childhood. This is contrary to what society believes. The reality is that my child's daily life would be affected by hospitalizations and all the associated unpleasantness, including nausea, pain, changes in appearance, and other ailments. The worst feeling as a parent is that of being powerless. Although I was supposed be a protector and caretaker, I couldn't help my child get relief. I could not make the pain go away or make it better. I could not erase the evil so my child could play.

It has taught me that it is not worth nagging or fighting about the little things in life like loading the dishwasher or hanging up the backpack after he comes home from school. It's about focusing on what is important in life. I want to show my child how to treat others, how to love unconditionally and that sharing joy is twice the joy. It may sound cliché and corny, but it is true. I realized that I don't want to waste my time on bickering and nagging, which won't improve my relationships with others or my quality of life.

In the beginning, I didn't have the energy or the strength to consider the feelings of others than myself and my child. Because my patience was nonexistent and my jealousy was immense, I was able to squabble with people about the smallest, most trivial things. I was jealous of my parents who didn't have to go through the same thing we did. They could continue living their lives as normal. It was so unfair. However, I quickly realized that there was so much love and support around us from all corners. We were able to overcome our difficulties because so many people showed empathy and support.

How has the experience of your child with cancer influenced your outlook on life?

Where do I begin? The shortness and fragility of life is a fact. In a matter of seconds, everything you have taken for granted can be destroyed or made obsolete. As of Marcus' diagnosis on 9 June 2015, I no longer consider anything in my life to be a given. Enjoy every moment and every second of it as if it were perfect!

You will be amazed at how much happiness you can bring to the lives of others if you show love and compassion. Realize that negativity is not as important as watching your children suffer and not being in a position to change it. My life has made the biggest difference by focusing my energy where it matters most.

I realized how insignificant and small I was in the world. But I also realized how important and loved I am to my family.

What has changed in your parenting?

I am aware that I was more relaxed in the beginning stages (about my expectations and "rules") and walked around doing a lot of things just because it was so miserable. As a parent, I shouldn't have to nag my child or hear negative comments about him. He already has so much to deal with and endure.

That thought made me feel a lot better. My child will make it through and be an adult. I did my part to raise him well. He will continue to grow up as a person with good morals, good values and good character. Soon, I realized there was no point in tiptoeing and took off the silk gloves. I tried my best to give him the food he wanted and entertainment that would make his life easier.

However, I did not stop making demands of him and encouraged him to strive to be the best he could in all areas, including school, health, and attitudes toward others.

If you look deeper, my parenting style has not changed. However, I have come to appreciate those moments when things go as I want.

No matter how prepared or experienced you might be, it's never easy to face a life-threatening, serious situation. It is important to not lose your self-control or allow it to overwhelm you. You can receive support and love during difficult times, and you can find joy in the moments that can give you the energy and strength to deal with any hardships.

Focus on the important things and keep your eyes focused. This includes your child's journey to recovery and the love between you and your family. When you feel helpless, hopeless, or overwhelmed by your grief, the security that surrounds you can be your friend. This is when you need to rely on the love around you to keep your feet on the ground.

This will forever change me as a person and my child as a parent. But, we chose to view it as a life lesson. It is an experience that will teach us how to spend our time here on Earth.

My Notes

CHAPTER NINE

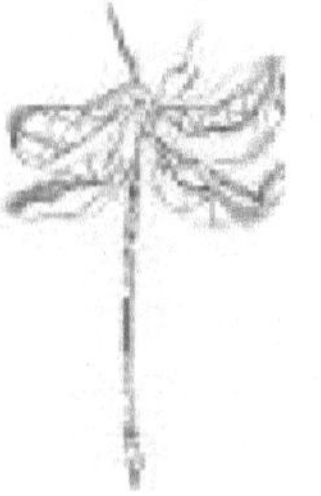

Escaping To Home

"Trotzdem Ja zum Leben sagan" means "Yes to living despite all."

– Jurriaan Kamp

As we neared the departure date, it became more stressful. We were due to begin another round of chemotherapy in the next few days.

Sweden on the 1st June. We were then expected to arrive at ward Q84 on the oncology floor of Astrid Lindgren Children's Hospital, Stockholm. Yousef needed to be strong enough for the long journey. The German staff made sure that this was possible. We were worried that Yousef would not be able to leave the hospital after so many setbacks. Yousef's passport was set to expire May 26th! It felt like we were illegal immigrants trying deceive authorities without proper paperwork. We had to cross borders with a stranger man we paid to smuggle in. (Learn more about this in a moment!)

There was tension and action: would it be possible to make it in the time allowed or would Yousef's passport run out? We needed to be in Sweden by the 28th May to settle things before reporting on Q84. It was very close! We couldn't afford to lose time, so Yousef would be back.

We had many details to remember before we could leave. I was responsible for ensuring that all paperwork was correct for both the country and the hospital. It was such a relief to find out that Yousef's situation had been thoroughly researched and was well-known by all the doctors. His case was handled by a team of specialists, including surgeons and oncologists. It was worth the hardship to be admitted at Astrid Lindgren Children's Hospital. It felt like we were in a bind between death and life. Then, we were told that we could come. I thought, my child can now come to my country. It was different than getting the permission to travel to Germany. This was my home, where I was born and where my son was a citizen. It was like a homecoming.

The Kinder Klinikum's nurses and doctors tried to make Yousef able to travel all this time. He was still at the hospital on May 22nd and had to be given platelets on May 25th. Because he had reacted badly to blood transfusions in the past, they administered medication to make his body accept platelets. This prevented him from becoming sick and forced us to delay the trip. It was clear that it would be difficult. To get to the new hospital, it would take 24 hours of driving. We would travel through Belgium, Holland and Denmark to reach the new hospital. Then we would continue on to Sweden. It is possible that some hospital staff thought it was crazy to attempt it.

My husband said that his uncles would drive us on the long journey.

I waited patiently for them to arrive that morning. Finally, I called my husband.

"Samer! Where are your uncles?" I inquired.

He said, "They aren't coming.".
"What? "What?!" I couldn't believe what was happening. He said, "Don't worry," "I found another person." Who? "I asked.

Samer had met a German man and reached out to him without my knowledge. His mother donated money to help pay for the guy and his camper van, which would take us all the way from Germany to Sweden. Samer believed the camper would make Yousef feel the most comfortable in his cast. And Yousef has always wanted to travel in a camper so Samer agreed. We didn't know the driver and I didn't like the idea of spending 24 hour in a van with a sick kid and a man I had never met.

"With a total stranger?" "Yes!" I replied.

"Don't worry!" Samer said.
We met the driver at the station, loaded our campervans and headed out. Yousef was excited to go and both of us felt like we were on a mission. Yousef went to sleep, while I stayed awake. I couldn't stop thinking. I didn't even speak to the driver, I was just desperate to get to Stockholm.

Since Yousef was about to lose his papers, I felt like I was a fugitive and that Wesef was being driven by someone who had been paid to smuggle me across borders. Were we going to be stopped? Were Yousef ill and would we have to stop? This would be a problem as we'd have to travel with an expired passport. To make sure he didn't get sick, I had mapped every hospital along the route so that we would know where to stop.

I had no idea what was going to happen. It felt like I was fleeing and trying to escape into my country!

The driver was committed to the mission. Poor driver only stopped driving when absolutely necessary - he drove almost continuously for 24 hours. He took a nap on the ferry to Denmark once, and then asked if I would mind if he rested for another 30-40 minutes. His stamina was amazing for a professional driver!

Many of our family and friends stayed up late to keep an eye on us throughout the night. We kept in touch with each other, texting back and forth all night, no one sleeping, everyone eager to hear that we had crossed over and are now safely in Sweden.

Because Yousef couldn't sleep, the camper was uncomfortable. It would have been much more comfortable to ride in a station wagon!

The morning of the 27th, driving across the bridge between Copenhagen and Malmo, will remain in my heart forever. It was a beautiful day with the sun rising over fields of yellow, like grapeseed. It felt like freedom. We didn't have to worry about getting stopped or having our passports stolen. We were free. We were free. We were thrilled to finally reach Stockholm, where we could visit my step-father and step-mother.

We would have liked a different welcome, but my father and Runa were anxious about our arrival. It was also felt by Yousef. It wasn't our house, it was my father's. I missed my mother so very much during that time. A mother is always a mom. Even if she only had a shoebox, I think my children and myself would have been welcomed. It doesn't matter if someone does it rightly or wrongly, but I would have done it differently. To my child, I would have said "I'm here for you." You can stay as long as it takes, this is your home." Perhaps I'm used to the Mediterranean culture and Arabic culture that focuses on close-knit families. There is so much connection. My dad and his wife were worried about Yousef's health; they were afraid he would die.

The Erbprinz hotel in Germany was like a family to us. They made us feel at home and took care of us. That was something I will never forget.

Yousef visited the hospital the next day. It's an old building that has so much character. The ward upstairs was open to us. Although it felt child-friendly, I was able to see him in the waiting area looking out at the park across the street, and watching the children playing football.

He said, "I can't get enough of playing football.".
"Yes, you'll be soon," I replied, believing that it would happen one day.

The doctors greeted us and told us all about the week ahead. The fifth round of chemotherapy for Yousef would start immediately, and the surgery would take place five weeks later. Because he was not well enough to continue on the schedule, it had to be delayed. My dad's wife prepared Swedish meatballs that night, when we returned home. They were a hit with Yousef. He was very hungry and had not eaten meat in many months.

I was required to sign in at the immigration office the next day. Yoursef's immune system was not strong enough to deal with all those who were waiting. His treatment was to start on Monday. He couldn't afford to be around all the germs. I went to immigration and was told that the wait time could be many hours. Yousef waited in the car alongside my father. After waiting for quite some time, I finally asked my father if it was possible to make it faster as I had a sick child outside. It took almost two hours. I asked the immigration officer if he would be able to come to my car and see my son when it was my turn. It wasn't something I would normally ask for, so I was thankful that he agreed to visit my son. He knew Yousef could not risk getting sick. It was a relief. Now we were "in the system". I could finally stop holding my breath.

Sunday was our first day at the hospital. The next morning, Yousef received anti-nausea medications before any treatment began. It was still a bit more severe than in Germany, but he did not get sick as much. Yousef felt so well that he was able to walk down to the playground. He was delighted to find that there was so much to do in Sweden, as opposed with Germany's hospital.

The Swedish approach to chemotherapy was quite different from what we are used to. To prevent sickness, the child is given anti-nausea medication before and after treatment. He can eat any food he likes and can tolerate. They didn't expect us to handle any of the chemotherapy at home. Instead, they kept Yousef at the hospital until he was able to go home. It was very child-friendly and he didn't need to take antibiotics every day. It was great to have Yousef's support. Friday 12 June was the day I began to write in my diary.

Because I feel helpless, I cry every time I look at Yousef. It's impossible for me to make it easier on him. Is there anything else? He woke up today with his nose bleeding. He had to have a hearing check. He was angry and depressed. He cried and feared for his cast being removed. His shoulders were in spasms because he was so stressed. They tried to calm him to make sure he was okay to go to the cast. But he wouldn't listen. He was left alone that night after they gave him painkillers to his neck.

It was a lot of work to reach Sweden. Because of the high doses of chemotherapy drugs, Yousef had to have his heart monitored. Because his red cell count was low, he had to be closely monitored in the event that he needed a blood transfusion. I was also confronted by the reality of the surgery. "What is it going to take for Yousef's body strength?"

I used to watch him sleeping, his legs crossed over my head. Every day, my sweet little boy went through so much. Not only did he have all the side effects of chemotherapy, but he also had a broken leg, sores on his leg, and blisters on the back of the foot from the cast. He had to be fasted every time they needed to open or repair his cast. From the moment his leg was cut in Germany, he was still traumatized.

Bright spots were highlighted when Johanna, my niece, and her family visited us. It was a joy for Yousef to be able to visit her family, especially her son Wilhelm, who was only a little over one year old. He made Yousef smile and laugh from the heart.

The Astrid Lindgren Children's Hospital was quite different from the

Kinder Klinikum in Germany. The children were entertained by Disney characters. Volunteers offered music and arts and crafts. The common kitchen was where everyone could eat together. To help families get through difficult times, they had professional clowns that would entertain them. My father loved the clowns, too!

Children could also collect beads from Childhood Cancer Foundation. Each child would receive a string and a bag made by them. Each child would receive a bead at the beginning of treatment and another for each injection, blood test or infusion. This long strand is now Yoursef.

He said, "Look at how many shots I took," one day. This is actually a good memory that's symbolic of everything he's been through.

We spent June in and out the hospital - Yousef was in treatment or trying get stronger enough to go on. My daughter and her friends visited us, and we had planned to visit my sister in North Carolina, but we ended up going back to the hospital. Yousef was unable to enjoy many of the things I planned. He missed visits from family and friends that he couldn't enjoy. A

4th-of- July party my oldest friend hosted for him. Cissi made him another barbeque a week later after he felt better!

On the 8th of Juli, we finally returned home. We had the apartment all to ourselves because Runa and my father were gone. Yousef, his sister Nathalie, and her friend were so happy to be laying on the sofa with them. These little moments of joy are priceless.

Yousef grew stronger and it was time for him to have his operation. Finally, we got to meet Dr. Otte. He was honest with us and didn't mince words. He is confident and direct, but not unkind.

"Will you ever let me play football again?" Yousef asked.

Dr. Otte stated, "No," but that "you could be a referee."

The doctor was confident in himself and I felt the same. I knew That Yousef also believed in me. He explained to us the preparations for the surgery which would be performed right away.

Yousef received injections five days prior to the operation to increase his white blood cells count. To make him strong enough to undergo the surgery, they had to build him up. He was excited about the surgery by this point. He wanted to remove the tumor and have his "new leg". The night before, he wasn't anxious, but he was happy and ready to go the next day. He woke up in the morning with some anxiety in his eyes. He was still excited to get out of bed, despite his nervousness.

MINDFUL BREATHING

When we understand that happiness is a choice and sadness is a decision, anger is a decision, and love is a option, then we can attain enlightenment.

— Brendan Burchard

Between the hurt you feel and how you react to it is a breath. You have all you need to alter your outcome.

You might not like what you get today. You might find yourself in a difficult situation. You might be thrown off your feet by the conversation that you have or the harsh words spoken by someone because they are stressed. Your choice. You have to decide what to do, how you should respond and how to remain calm in the face of the storm.

Breathe. This small breath is more powerful than the raging winds and the storm. Make sure you use it.

Breath is vital. William Atkinson

My Notes

CHAPTER TEN

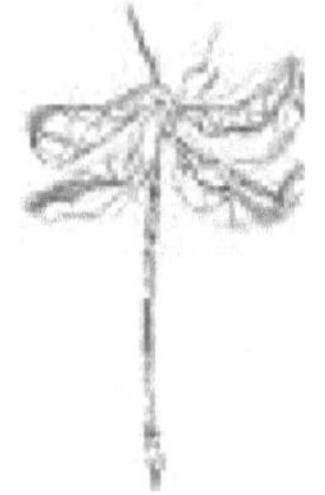

I See The Future

"Life cannot be understood backwards. It must be lived forwards."

– Søren Kierkegaard

A Five minutes before 8:00 on the 15th July, the day of surgery, I hadn't spoken to the surgeon. By this point, we were supposed to be heading down to the operating area. About a quarter of an hour later, Dr. Otte finally came in. He was calm and answered some of my questions. Finally, we were taken to the operating room. The entire team was waiting for Yousef when we arrived.

All of the equipment was extremely clean, which is important for any type of orthopedic surgery. When he saw the spacious, clean operating room, Yousef smiled. He was then wheeled into the room and moved to the table with a special, heated, inflated mattress. I was allowed to go with him but told to avoid all covered instruments.

I stood there, looking at the people preparing. I asked Yousef.

What are you going to be dreaming about right now? Imagine that you're going to bed and have a dream. When you wake up, I'll be right there beside you.

Before we told the Trouble Tree story, we talked about the field that we often go to. He also mentioned his German Shepherd, which he hopes to have one day.

An anesthesiologist arrived and was ready to put Yousef into sleep. Yousef looked happy and calm. He fell asleep quickly after the medicine was administered to his IV.

"Sweet dreams Yousef," I whispered.

I took a picture of him, sleeping. I kept my composure even though I felt emotional. I wanted to stay positive for him, so he wouldn't pick up negative feelings from me and get scared. Two nurses came over and walked me out. I understand that sometimes parents have a hard time leaving their child. They might faint, or make a scene.

"Thank you," they said to me.

"Why?"

"For making it easy for us. When a child is calm or just falls asleep, it is so much easier."

I left the hospital to walk on the grounds of the lovely Haga Parken – the national park right across from the hospital. It is the home of our royal Princess, and a place I had come to many times before. This is the park I used to walk in, and I did my normal route. The green all around me, the blue sky, it was warm, not hot – a pleasant day, with shady trees. I marveled at the

Swedish summer, how different it was from the desert where I've lived for twenty-five years.

I appreciated the smell of the earth, the sound of the birds. It was very empty, early in the morning in the middle of the week. I looked over the field, remembering when I brought my girls here when they were small: 8 and 2 years old. It was December, and the park was full of snow. Twenty years ago, I had been in this same place sledding with my two small daughters – never imagining I'd be here today, waiting for my young son.

I walked quite a while, knowing the operation would take some time. I let myself feel the sun and warm breeze touch my face, allowing myself to breathe. I sat on a bench overlooking a slope that led down to a green field. It reminded me of the Trouble Tree story Yousef asks for: a tranquil place, with trees to hang your worries. I was very worry-free this morning, in spite of the fact my child was in surgery. Nature is so healing. I just sat and listened to the birds and the leaves rattling in the wind. It was so calming. I had a feeling of trust and faith that everything would be alright.

On this same day in London, my younger daughter Nathalie was graduating from London College of Fashion, and I wasn't there with her. She had done really well and was an Honors student. I know it was hard for her. Not only was her mother not with her, but her little brother was having a huge operation to save his leg and his life. She was celebrating, and her brother was going through all this.

"Please, baby, go and enjoy your day," I said. I was relieved that her father was with her, so she wasn't alone, and she sent me pictures from her day.

I walked to the other side of the park and sat down on a bench and looked out. Across from me, down in the field, I saw a blond young man with his German Shepherd by his side.

Just before falling asleep, Yousef had spoken about a field where he was going to be with his German Shepherd – and here it was, that very scene. Like a snapshot of the future – a picture of Yousef as a young man, grown up and completely healed and well after all this, enjoying his life out in the sunshine with his beloved dog. I prayed it would be so.

The doctor called me around 11:00 am, two and a half hours after I'd left Yousef's side. I was a little surprised because I thought it might take the whole day. He told me to wait an hour or so, and then Yousef would be in recovery, and I would be able to see him.

When I returned to the hospital, I was shocked by what I saw. Yousef was so pale; he'd lost a lot of blood, and his leg was still bleeding. He had to stay in the recovery area for a couple of hours as the blood had to drain. He had a nerve block for his leg, otherwise, the pain would have been excruciating. You can imagine cutting and drilling into a bone. Even days later, they were giving him all sorts of medicines just to keep him out of pain. Yousef didn't do well; he was actually horrible on morphine – it affected his mood, his personality.

"Go away, I want to kill you!" he said to me one day in a voice I didn't even recognize.

For the next five days, I stayed next to him. On the 19th, his sister Salina came to visit with her husband, Liam, which meant I got a little bit of a break. Yousef wasn't feeling very well and wasn't very friendly toward his sister and brother-in-law. Liam helped a lot because he was patient and calm. Salina and Liam had rented an apartment, thinking that maybe, we could come and stay with them, but of course, it was too soon. Yousef wasn't doing well enough to leave the hospital.

Nathalie also came to see Yousef, and so did her dad, my ex-husband. Under the pain, Yousef did seem glad to have everyone there. I wish he could have enjoyed it more. For me, it meant I had a chance to go outside for a coffee by myself, to have a moment alone, away from Yousef's bedside. I also had the support of my daughters, which was so wonderful. They would listen and were very encouraging. My daughters would cook in the kitchen outside the ward, and Salina even baked pies and brought them to us. It was amazing to have home-cooked food after all this time.

I thought it was OK for me to leave Yousef for brief stretches of time, but, once when Nathalie was with him, he didn't feel comfortable telling her had to go to the bathroom. He wound up sitting in the mess until the next day, too embarrassed to tell anyone. The nurses helped us to take care of it, and I told him not to be ashamed. I realized I couldn't take more than a short time away from him.

Immediately after the surgery, Yousef was supposed to start moving his leg. He couldn't put any pressure on it yet, but the nurses and physiotherapists would come and try to begin exercising it to help the healing. They couldn't let it drop or lower it all the way to the floor yet. Yousef would scream no matter how careful they were or how slowly they moved him.

It was ten days after the surgery before Yousef moved to a wheelchair and the therapists slowly started to lower his leg to the floor. He looked so weak and yellow. It would still be some time before he could stand, but this was a big step. Once he was in the wheelchair, we could take him outside. One day we all played outside, and even Yousef had fun and enjoyed some ice cream. On other days, he wasn't doing well at all. On the Sunday before Salina and Liam were to leave, we planned to have big celebration brunch in the park where I'd walked the day of the surgery. We were all looking forward to it so much, but Yousef didn't feel well enough to go, and I didn't want to leave him.

Salina and Liam spoiled us while they were there. They bought us an espresso machine and a TV and told us that we would have our own home soon. It was sad to see them go. Right after they left, Yousef moved to Q84, the oncology floor, to prepare for his next round of chemo. It was only 11 days after his operation. I wondered how he would manage it.

I know we have a choice about how to feel, even when things are difficult. I kept telling myself that I can choose to be happy during this difficult time. It was important to keep asking the question, 'What can I do to make it better?' I chose to take it one moment at a time and to be the best possible mother to Yousef I could be, in each moment. In order to do that, I had to be as clear as I could about my own thoughts and feelings.

We were alone together again. We had a routine: I'd make breakfast, we'd watch a couple of TV shows in the morning, sitting together in the bed. Then he'd go to physiotherapy. In the beginning, he would scream like crazy, but it got better over time. He started to enjoy arts and crafts, and it kept him busy. He started to crave all sorts of food because he could have whatever he wanted, and his appetite was back. He asked for cake, which he loves. I was glad I could cook for him in the kitchen on Q84.

At the "Lekterapin," the activity center, the children are free to express themselves in so many ways, and now that Yousef was feeling better, he could enjoy it. The people who work there are all truly wonderful, so caring and giving. They make the hospital stay a little easier for the children, siblings, and parents.

At Astrid Lindgren, they've also thought of the children who can't go down to the Lekterapin because they're having chemo. They have a team called "Pysselbyrån" (Arts & Crafts) who would come around to us. I used to look forward to them because they came smiling, with themes and activities for adults and children alike. They were a distraction from the routine that you learn to accept as the new reality. Arts and crafts, play, and music therapy – they all help to give your child (and you) a break. Maybe it also helps everyone to emotionally process what's going on.

On the 31st of July, Yousef stood up for the first time. He had tears streaming down his cheeks. He was elated, screaming from pain and excitement. I have a picture from that day. This moment was a confirmation to him that he would be able to use his leg again. It had been 5 months and 7 days since he had last stood. When he was recently asked what it felt like to be able to stand up again on his own two legs, all he said was, "Amazing."

How does it get any better than that?

After physio that day, we went upstairs to the ward, and he wanted to sit in the living room! Then on his own, he wheeled himself to the examination room where his favorite nurse, Christopher, gave him his injection and medicines. Christopher told me afterward that he took them easily.

Yousef came back out to the living room to do some activity as "pyssel byrån," (arts and crafts,) had come. He made a beautiful painting. Then we left the hospital and came home. That night, before falling asleep, he read a whole chapter in his new book, The Mystery of the Griefer's Mark- a Mine Craft book.

Wow what a day, I thought. I was so happy for him. What if tomorrow could be an even better day? What else is possible?

At the end of July, things were looking much better. I was excited to write my diary entry for Thursday 30 July 2015,

What a day today has been! This morning, Yousef woke up in a really good mood. He started writing today's schedule then had his breakfast. At 9.30 am he had his heart test, which was good. Then he came back to the room and slept for over an hour.

At 1:00 pm we had an appointment with the Physio. There, Yousef played the Wii game "Mario Kart " while one of the Physiotherapist lowered his leg. It was down on the floor for 10 minutes! Afterward, he moved over to the barre where he was able to stand up, holding on while they managed to lower his leg all the way down to the floor. He stood on both legs for 5 minutes!

Such simple things, and so amazing!

I've written a bit about getting support, and I really believe having people you can rely on is so important. There were psychologists we could have spoken to, and I am sure they are very useful to some people. When we were in Germany, a psychologist came to see Yousef, but she had an approach that didn't work. Yousef refused to speak with her every time she came. When we got to Sweden, the psychologist had a different approach, and she accepted that Yousef didn't want to talk. Instead, Yousef was offered music therapy, and he later met Andreas in the "Lekterapin." He and Andreas connected – and he taught Yousef to create his own music.

There was also a woman who made films with the children, and Yousef loved that. They used an app on the iPad, and Yousef used his own Legos, which are his favorite toys. When I watched him, I thought even if he has missed almost a year of school, he's learned so many other things this year.

Worry pretends to be necessary, but serves no purpose."

— Eckhardt Tolle

Sometimes, our mind runs away with us. Off we go, and now, we aren't free, we are captive. We aren't able to be present with others. We don't have space in our hearts for care or listening. Our minds are racing, and it takes up all the room in our hearts that we need for other things. Now is not the time to allow worry to drag us away. Let worry go on its way, alone. Watch it, like a cloud slips from your view...like a wave recedes back into the ocean.

Whenever you are getting carried away with worry, close your eyes for a moment.

Imagine you are holding a piece of chalk in your hand.

See a chalkboard in front of you.

Begin writing numbers down, as if you are making a list.

1.

2.

3.

et

c.

Now, see yourself writing down the first thing that is bothering you – the worst thing. Condense it down to a few words, or maybe just one word.

Now, watch your other hand as it picks up an eraser or a rag. Erase the worry. Go over each letter until there isn't a trace to be seen of the words you've written about your worry or concern.

When the worry has been entirely wiped away, go on to number 2. In your mind's eye, see yourself write the next concern. Again, condense it to just a few words. Now, pick up the eraser and wipe it completely away.

Do this for each and every worry you have: letting your mind acknowledge and then erase and release them.

You can do this exercise to help you relax or to fall asleep at night, too. It comes from a hypnosis technique.

To use it for that purpose, see yourself writing numbers from 10 down to 1, erasing them as you go.

For example:

In your mind's eye, see your hand writing the number "10."

Then, see your hand erasing the number "10" completely.

Watch your hand writing number "9." Imagine erasing "9", and so on.

My Notes

CHAPTER ELEVEN

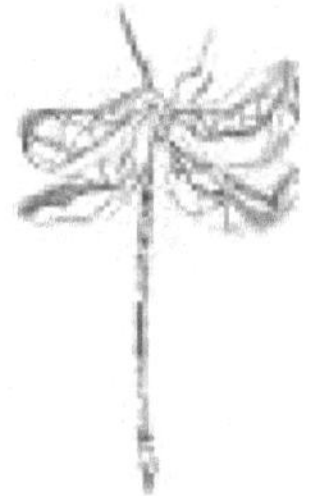

Now I Have More Time

You will never have this day with your children again. Tomorrow they will be a little older than they were today. This day is a gift."

– Sutton Coldfield

One day, Yousef asked me, ""How do you get cancer?"

"I don't know. Let's ask the doctor," I said.

So when he came up from his next Physio appointment, he did. It was a doctor he said he didn't like just a few days before. I don't know if he was satisfied with her answer.

"No one knows for sure," she said.

"Can you get more cancers?" he asked.

"Sadly, yes," she said.

The doctor told Yousef she was very happy he was asking questions, she said he could ask anytime, through me, or directly.

It was natural for him to wonder about it for himself, but he had also just seen his friend Justin experience a recurrence of leukemia. Justin had been doing well after treatment, and just as everyone thought he was in the clear, he got sick again.

As I write this, Justin is recovering from having a bone marrow transplant. As soon as he is well enough for visitors, Yousef wants to go and see him.

Yousef has seen and experienced too much for his years. He also knows that his grandmother is dying of cancer. There is a lot of illness around him. I would love him never to have to wonder about getting sick again or dying prematurely. But, he is reminded of his condition all the time, and he will be checked and treated for years to come. I tell him that no one is promised a certain number of years – at any moment, any one of us might die from cancer or something else. It's a lesson that many adults don't even understand, and my nine-year-old was confronted with it every day. As for me, I feel blessed that, now, I have more time with Yousef. Anything could happen to anyone, any day. I am now with him, and I appreciate every moment.

Astrid Lindgren Children's Hospital had many things to keep our spirits up, and not just for the patients and parents. There was a woman who ran activities for the young siblings of the patients because they need attention, too. She baked each morning for all of us. We'd wake up to the good smell of vanilla and cinnamon. One day, there was a band on the oncology floor – and of course, there were clowns! It was such a healing environment, very positive and child-friendly. When we were there, it felt very supportive, very good.

Going home to my father's apartment, however, was another story. Just getting into the apartment was a challenge. They live up a flight of stairs, and I would have to carry Yousef up, then go back down and carry up the wheelchair. I don't know where I got the strength from – it's incredible how you can do anything when you just focus on it.

Yousef used to hug me and say, "I love you, Mamma! Thank you for taking care of me!"

That gave me even more strength. Only later did a driver tell me there was a stair climber in some of the wheelchair taxis.

"No one mentioned it to you?" he asked.

"No, I didn't know you could even ask for such a thing."

My father apologized that he couldn't help more. Living at his apartment was a challenge in other ways. He and Runa were set in their ways, and I felt we were in their way, interrupting their routine. I appreciated their support and was grateful when my father tried to joke with Yousef, even if he was surly in his reply sometimes because he wasn't feeling well.

Things were complicated in more ways than that. When Yousef started school in September, he was still under treatment. Imagine having to start a new school (not just a new school *year*) sick from chemo and still recovering from surgery! Plus, we had just moved into our own apartment. Yousef could now stand on his crutches, but he became exhausted if he had to walk too far or stand for too long. He was happy that day.

Yousef found that school in Sweden is different from Dubai. Here, students have hot lunch and breakfast and fruit during the day for snacks. Yousef stays after school for junior club where he takes part in different activities such as "Home Ec." He has a snack and an after-school program called "Research and Development," which is supervised time to do homework. In Dubai, you bring your own lunch, pay for extracurricular activities, and there is no time after school to do your homework with supervision! But Yousef had to learn to deal with how his peers would react to him. I don't know what makes kids so cruel sometimes, but Yousef, sadly, had to deal with bullying in his new school, right alongside everything else.

Sometimes, I watch Yousef hopping around on his leg, and I am amazed by how well he has adjusted and how happy he is most of the time. Salina has reflected on how Yousef is now: open, and able to communicate easily with me. He might be moody, but he is getting into his teen years, so it might be perfectly normal, not related at all to after-effects of treatment or his physical condition – just puberty!

For Yousef, the whole experience was about more than the illness, treatment, or even the surgery. There was the shock of breaking his leg during his favorite activity at school and having to accept that he would never play football again. Then he was torn away from his childhood home and country, his school, and his friends. He was separated from his father, brother, and sisters. He had to live in Germany - a foreign country with a different language then move again for surgery, which was terrifying all by itself. – He had visited my family in Sweden before but had never lived there. I can't tell you how hard it was adjusting to the ways of a different hospital where the routines and attitude were so different from the Kinder Klinikum in Germany.

You don't realize that you enter a culture – a way to practice medicine that is unique to that hospital. Leaving it means you take your disease, at whatever stage, and you enter a whole new culture and have to learn how it works. You miss some of the things from the last place – even though you'd never choose in a million years to be in either one.

Yousef is still adjusting to the after-effects of his surgery and the new reality of his body now. That's a lot for a little boy. Recently, he wrote an essay for school. The actual assignment was to imagine having to leave your home because of war – becoming a refugee, forced to leave your friends and family because of violence. But Yousef wrote it from his personal experience.

"I don't have to imagine war," he said, "I had to leave my home and friends and school."

I agreed. Look at the language we use about cancer: we fight it, or it's called a battle for your life, and we want to "beat it." Yousef didn't have to imagine being a refugee because of a war.

Awareness

If you could be calm and centered whenever you had to explain something to your child, or when you ask some questions of the doctor, how would that help?

If you could become mindful and aware of something soothing or beautiful in your surroundings once (or more) per day- what might be different?

A Practice to Try:

Become conscious of the room you are in. Locate something that looks beautiful or attractive to you. Maybe you can look at a window, at trees, or the sky.

Or, find something that gives you a sense of love or peace.

Become aware of the beauty, love, or peace. Focus on it.

Breathe.

Say, "And now I am fully here. Not in the future or the past. Right here and right now. Hear clearly. I ask for what I need, right now, in this moment." Breathe.

My Notes

CHAPTER TWELVE

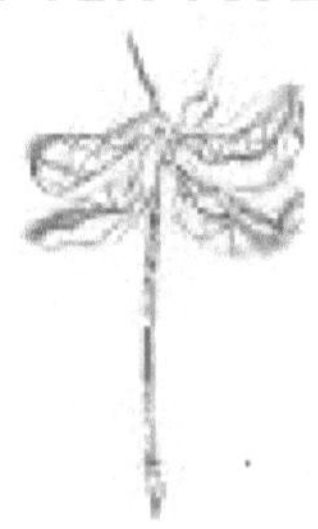

Inspiring Friends

"I never met a bitter person who was thankful. Or a thankful person who was bitter."

— Nick Vujicic

We are never the same after cancer. Not as individuals, or as a family. Plenty of times, cancer doesn't kill the patient, but it can definitely kill marriages, cause rifts in families, and breaks between friends. Cancer shows us how fear brings out the worst in people. For example, at school Yousef experienced bullying – with one child threatening to kick him in the leg; even telling him, "I hope you get the cancer back!" What makes a child say something like that? It didn't seem there was anything personal between them, no animosity, no fight. But kids can be so cruel – and I think it was out of fear. Yousef walked a little differently, and he started school in a wheelchair, and it made him the target of a bully. And we all know bullies are children (and adults) who have been picked on and feel inadequate themselves.

Cancer can open our eyes, too. We see the job, or the life we had wasn't worth all the lifetime we were devoting to it. We realize: nobody is promised tomorrow, and now is the time to live the life we dreamed of. Sometimes that means leaving jobs or lifestyles or relationships. It can mean we finally get the courage to pursue our dreams. Cancer changes us and everything around us, and sometimes, if we are intentional about it, it can change our lives for the better. We figure out that now is the time to appreciate the people we love and do and say what is in our hearts.

"What would you like people to know about what you've been through?" I asked Yousef recently.

"How it is to sit in bed all day long with nothing to do – so people know that there are people in the world who can't do anything but sit and wait," Yousef said. He learned empathy, and he wanted to teach that to others.

"People will know what I've been through, and what others are going through," he said.

My friend Shaikha lost her arm to cancer when she was only two. Shaikha is an inspiration. She says people who stare or judge her are "silly." She knows it is a prejudice that comes from fear. She says, yes, she is different, meaning unique, unlike the ordinary rest of the world. She is a living example of self-acceptance and courage. I asked her what she would tell a child and his or her parents about the lasting effects of cancer, particularly when their bodies look or work differently afterward.

Me: You were very young when you lost your arm, but it impacted the rest of your life in ways that most of us cannot imagine. What would you like us to know about you?

- At the beginning, I was always upset about being different from other kids. I was not accepted by the children around me, and they used to tease me about my prosthetic arm. I realized that wearing it does not add anything to me. It just makes people think that I look like them. Eventually, I decided to step up and face my life without wearing it.

What would you tell a child who worries that they will be "different" after their illness?

- I'd tell them don't feel "different," feel special because you are special and unique. Most of the people out there are alike, yet God has chosen us to look unique and special.

What encouragement or words of wisdom would you give to parents about how to cope with the physical changes their child might experience?

- Stay strong. Being upset about something that took place will not change the fact of the disease, or (in my case) the limb the child lost. Feeling sorry or looking at him with pity will not make him stronger. The damage is done. Work together to make the child more confident, let him be independent, let him try and fail. The more he tries, the better he will be. When kids in school make fun of the child, teach him how to respond and act. Don't feel sorry, or go down to the school to handle it for him. That makes him feel weaker. Teach him to survive without you. By doing too much for the child, he will never learn he can do it himself, which is not right in my opinion. They need to learn the hard way to succeed in their life. They need to make the child proud of how he looks and who he is. Do not look at your child with pity all the time.

What did your own parents do RIGHT? What would you have preferred they do differently?

- My parents, God bless them, were the exact opposite. My dad was overprotective and always feels sorry for me and thinks that I need help in every single thing I do. My mum made me not feel any different in anything. She never treated me differently even when I could not handle things like tying my hair, carrying things, drawing lines on the notebook. However, she wasn't mean, she just made me learn how to handle things on my own and to figure out a way to do things without anyone's help. It takes a brave mum to do that for her child, especially after all the medical treatments the child has gone through. But, here I am standing in front of the world proud of who I am, where I am, and how I look. A huge "thank you" goes to my mother who suffered by raising me to make me who I am now.

What would you say to a child, to encourage, console or inspire?

- Love yourself for who you are. Be proud of how you look. Feel that you're special. YOU ARE UNIQUE. Move on and try to inspire the world with what you can do. Listen, pick and choose what you hear from people. Turn the sentences that have a negative impact on you into a positive sentence. Remember, in spite of someone's silly words: YOU ARE UNIQUE.

You are so inspirational! What have people said to you about your attitude, belief, abilities?

- Believe it or not, I am very happy with the way I look and never want to wear a prosthetic. All it does is please people's eyes. I am here the way I am. I have accepted myself and love the way I look. I am living my life better than any normal person. Accept yourself, love yourself, believe in your capabilities. Disability is not when you have a missing limb, it's when you stop and limit yourself.

I understand not everyone has been kind to you. How do you handle their reactions? What would you say to a parent, or a child, who might find themselves facing some harsh or bullying experiences as a result of their illness?

- I am who I am. I have accepted how I look, now the world has to accept me. I give a huge smile, and I think twice before reacting. In the beginning, it's the parents who have to help the child accept what happened to them. The parent should make the child feel confident, even when people stare or point at them. If a parent is over-protective, the child is weaker in personality. Do speak to the child every now and then. Show him movies, real stories where people deal with disabilities or illness, so he can see it happens to others in the world. It will help the child develop the ability to build more confidence in themselves.

What have you learned about life, about others, and about yourself as a result of your different-ability?

- I have learned that life is not easy, but you can handle it with the right perspective. I learned that, in general, people will underestimate you regardless of your disability. That is human nature. But, YOU ARE THE SPECIAL ONE. You change the world by being yourself and doing all you are able to do. That will teach other people how to see you – you will show them what "different" means.

Sometimes I watch Yousef hopping around on his leg, and I am amazed by how well- adjusted and happy he is most of the time. He might get moody, but he is getting into his teen years, so it might be perfectly normal, not related at all to after-effects of treatment or his physical condition.

When we were in Germany, I heard about a man called Nicholas Vujicic, an Australian born with Tetra-Amelia Syndrome, a rare disorder characterized by the absence of arms and legs. Today, Nick is a motivational speaker and author of seven books. He writes about life, love, and selfacceptance. He writes about family, productivity, work, and the power of faith and standing strong. Despite suffering from bullying and struggling mentally and physically, he didn't give up.

I showed Yousef some of his YouTube videos. He was inspired how Nick was able to move without any legs and arms. And how he didn't give up. Yousef said,

"He inspired me by how he can go every day, and he makes jokes about himself, and he's always happy. He can do a lot of stuff."

I asked him what he learned from Nick, and he said,

"Try to be happy all the time."

Last year in October, Nick came to Stockholm. Yousef and I went to hear him speak, and we got a chance to meet him. It was an amazing experience for Yousef. Once again, he was shown that you can always do things if you believe you can, and it's okay if you don't make it right, you just try again. I have a picture of Yousef hugging Nick, which I just love. Nick says,

"... for every disability you have, you are blessed with more than enough abilities to overcome your challenges."

No, Nick couldn't hug Yousef back with his arms, but his attitude and what he taught Yousef was even better, more powerful, more lasting. He had the ability to more than overcome his challenges, and so does Yousef.

My Notes

CHAPTER THIRTEEN

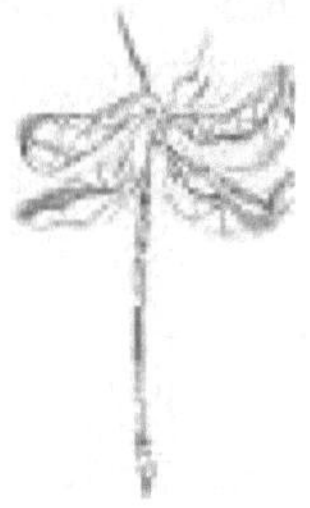

Fear Is a Dragon

"It is impossible to control your thoughts. They happen at the speed of light. But...the one thing you do have control over is how you react to the thought you just had."

— Trevor Blake

Yousef finished chemo at the end of November. On the day he was discharged, the doctor gave me all the paperwork and instructions for follow-ups. I had no idea what to expect.

"Oh my God!"

He handed me the plan for ten years' worth of follow-ups that would include check-ups every six weeks in the first year, then every three months in the second. He'd need blood work, chest X-rays, and X-rays of his leg. In addition, any time we planned to travel, he'd need a check-up first. All of this is just for the cancer, not the leg. For that, we have a whole different protocol!

Yousef's birthday is December 2nd, and his wish was to spend it back home in Dubai. We planned to go, but I knew we probably wouldn't be able to make it in time for his birthday. So I arranged for Salina, Liam, Jill, Ramsey, and Nathalie all to come home (to Sweden) that weekend to surprise him. He'd wanted that too: for everyone to be there for his birthday. When the doorbell rang, and they were all there, he couldn't believe his eyes!

We went to the museum together, Yousef in the wheelchair. He really enjoyed it. Then we had a combined party to celebrate both finishing his treatment and his birthday. While I'd planned the weekend, I'd been counting the days, thinking that he could very well be in the hospital, sick from the after-effects of his last round of chemo. Normally, this would have been the week when he'd be very weak and prone to complications. Yousef got lucky. He never had to go back into the hospital again. Yousef had learned that many times I couldn't keep promises because things out of our control would come up. We had an understanding. We would plan and go forward as if things would work out, but we would accept it if something happened to change our plans. He never questioned me.

We did get to Dubai later in December, although, right up to the last day I wasn't sure he'd be well enough to fly. The trip to Dubai was very emotional. Yousef was in compression socks for the plane and still in his difficult-tomanage wheelchair, and we were returning for the first time in nearly a year to where this journey had begun. We were not the same people, but he'd looked forward to it so much, and it was great for him to be there.

Salina had arranged a picnic at the beach, and our family and friends came. It was still a little cool in Dubai, but Yousef loved being in the sand. Dubai isn't as wheelchair-friendly as other parts of the world, so he had to move around more on his crutches, which was a boost for him – it gave him some independence. He had to use his leg a bit more, and he started believing in himself and in his leg. He saw that it was OK to use it. He knew there were stairs to get into our building before the elevator. We could carry him, but he practiced in order to do it by himself. He was able to visit his old school, and he stayed with his friends for a whole day. He still stays in touch with them through Skype and Minecraft. It seems those boys are in my house all the time through that technology.

We spent the New Year in Dubai and came back to Sweden in the middle of January. He'd missed a bit of school, but I thought that was alright under the circumstances, although, the school isn't always so happy when I keep him out for travel or whatever. We both feel school and education are important, but so is enjoying life, experiencing new things, and seeing family and friends. Cancer puts everything into perspective.

Yousef realizes he can't go back to Dubai to live, but the trip was reassuring. It's only a six-hour flight away. He might not be living there, but he can visit. Recently I asked him whether he wanted to go and live in Dubai again.

"No, I want to live in Sweden."

I don't know why he prefers it; maybe he realizes they don't have the treatment options for cancer in Dubai. His father has also told him that the doctors are better in Sweden. The hospital is familiar, and they take good care of him. He knows and trusts his surgeon. Maybe he feels safe here.

I know he thinks about things that he doesn't talk about. His friend Justin almost died of leukemia. He started his chemo much earlier than Yousef. He went through so much - he was in a coma for six weeks. When Justin finished up his treatment, everyone thought he was going to be fine. When he got sick again, it was such a shock to Yousef, and he was so upset. Justin became really depressed; he didn't want to live and fight anymore.

Justin's mother is afraid.

"What will it take for you to let that go?" I asked her.

"I am afraid to believe it's going to be OK," she said.

Of course, Yousef is aware of all this, but he doesn't talk about it.

When we came back from Dubai this year in January, my step-mother was back in hospital with cancer. We knew she was dying. That was when Yousef started asking whether you can get cancer again. I knew I had to be careful talking to him, not to upset him and add to his concerns.

Yousef is keeping his attitude up; he's not depressed, but no one knows what Methotrexate, one of his main chemo drug, does to the mind. It might cause anxiety or depression. They do a lot of follow-up on that, asking about his moods, thoughts, and effect. I asked the psychologist recently about some of his moodiness.

“Is it the Methotrexate or the after-effects of chemo in general – or is it puberty?!”

Nobody seems to know for sure. I’m going to look at him as a budding teenager and let it be.

When we were in Germany, and they first released Yousef to me between treatments, they sent me home with shots and pills and a strict schedule to follow to manage his nausea and counteract the chemo. They released us with stern warnings to watch his diet and look out for dangerous side effects. They sent me off all by myself, with a boy who was so sick. It was terrifying. I had a milder form of that same feeling when they signed us out of Q84 at Astrid Lindgren for the last time. I felt very much on my own. I am sure other patients and family members feel that way.

There is a study in Canada where they followed families after their children were released from cancer treatment. The effects on a family can be devastating, and the feeling of being completely alone once they are discharged from the hospital or from treatment is frightening and common. The study found that if the family is followed by a coach, after six months, the children and the whole family are doing much better than families without one. Coaching improves the outcome of long-term recovery and the health of the family system.

In my opinion, coaching can, at times, be more effective to deal with more things than psychotherapy. Psychologists focus on analyzing the source of fear, and they focus on the past. Coaching focuses on the now and on the future. It is positive and forward-looking. I’d much rather ask, “What do we do now? Here we are, a family, we are different now. We have a child who has gone through this difficult thing – and now, what?”

I believe you don’t go into the fear. Instead, you look at the possibilities. That is what coaching does. It’s like being confronted with a monster, say, a dragon. As a coach, I would say, “See your dragon (fear), and ask what can I do with that?”

Likewise, I don’t focus on what Yousef can’t do but what he CAN do. His surgeon, Dr. Otte has the same approach. When Yousef told him he wanted to play football, Dr. Otte said,

“What if you could be the referee?”

Our minds will limit everything unless we focus differently. There is life after cancer, and what you must focus on is *life*. I encourage Yousef to look at what he <u>will</u> be able to do – bicycle, or swim -- rather than what he cannot. I think about what happens to children after they are released from their treatment and rehabilitation. They don't have coaches; and through the long months of illness and debilitating chemo, they learn about limitation instead of possibility. What would it take to turn that around?

Three hundred kids each year used to be diagnosed with cancer in Sweden, and today that number has risen to 350 – every year. The population here is small, so that is a really big number. Survival rates are improving, and in the future, will get even better, but cancer isn't going away. The world isn't getting less toxic. How will we help those children to adjust to their new reality and make the most of everything they have experienced and learned?

Butterfly Hug

What might be possible if your body and mind were brought into alignment and peace, physiologically? This practice is called bilateral stimulation. It is said to balance the mind and body and to reduce anxiety. Here is how to do it:

Cross your arms over your chest as if you are hugging yourself. Put your hands on opposite biceps, like this:

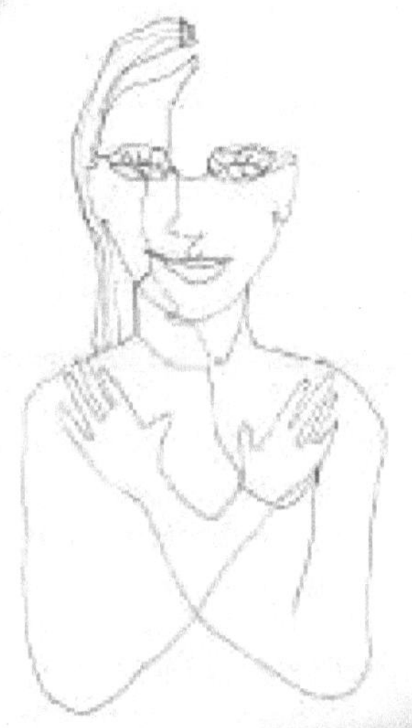

Slowly and gently tap, first one hand, then the other, on your arm.

Do this while you breathe in and out five times. Deep slow breaths.

You can teach your child to do the Butterfly Hug as well. It will give him or her a way to self-soothe whenever they need to.

AMANDA'S STORY

I interviewed Amanda Eriksson, who was a first-time mother when her threemonth-old daughter was diagnosed with cancer. I've translated their story from Swedish.

Helene: As a young new mother, hearing your baby is sick is just devastating. Can you give us just a couple of sentences that tell our readers what happened to your family? (What was the diagnosis, how did you find out your daughter was sick, what the treatment was?)

Estelle was born in September 2014. Around Christmas time, when she was 3 months old, she started getting a cold and had a fever on and off through January and February. She also had a severe cough and developed croup. We were in and out of the emergency room. She had bacteria in the urine all the time, but the doctors blamed it on the bacteria in the diaper. In the end, now early March, the nurse at our pediatric clinic sent us to get an ultrasound to see whether the bacteria had spread to the kidneys. They found a tumor larger than a tennis ball on Estelle's left kidney. When the doctor called and said they'd found something, I didn't know how serious it was. But two hours later, we were at the children's oncology ward, and that same evening they began chemotherapy. In the following ten months, Estelle went through surgery, radiation, and frequent chemotherapy treatments. She had clear cell sarcoma, a rare kidney tumor.

What did you do to try to mother your infant in normal ways? For example, I know you breastfed through chemo. Tell us about that. What else?

I breastfed Estelle throughout the treatment and continued even a few months afterward. I am so grateful that I had the opportunity to do this, and it made it easier for all needle sticks and check-ups. The best thing was to have my beloved daughter next to me and feel her breath and heart beating against me. The two of us became one and created the vital ties to heal each other's hearts.

We were living under very difficult circumstances and mostly isolated from other children and families, but the staff at the oncology ward Q84 were amazing, Pysselbyrån (Arts & Crafts) and Lekterapin (play-therapy center) were incredibly important for us. Even music became important. We brought Estelle's children songs with us, ones we've played since she was born. I remember how we danced every day in the room or in the kitchen of the ward. We sang a lot, laughed and hugged. We were always together, the three of us, we were and still are the strongest when we're together!

What was important for your self-care?

I lost myself completely during Estelle's treatment. I did not leave her for a second, even when I would take a shower, I took her into the bathroom. If we had anything to buy, my partner Calle had to go. Sometimes I forced myself to go out for a walk to get fresh air and leave the hospital walls. Haga Parken was an oasis. I walked around and cried and let everything go, and then filled myself with a new energy that gave me new strength and courage, I was recharged. I even wrote a diary, and it was liberating to get out all the feelings and experiences. And even now, in hindsight, it is nice to revisit.

Where did your support come from?

My beloved Calle, Estelle's father. We were each other's best friends in life's worst moments. As well as my family, some friends, and of course, all the fantastic hospital staff.

How are you a different parent than you might have been otherwise?

I wake up every day and thank the higher powers that Estelle is next to me. I am present in a totally different way, I do not stress and worry about the little things. I give Estelle all my time. I dare to say NO to things I do not want to do or feel I don't have the strength for. I am staying with my family's energy and mine.

Tell us how your daughter is now (people will want to read it for encouragement!)

Today, Estelle is 3 years old and is doing well. She is the world's most wonderful, empathetic, and precocious girl! She feels much wiser - beyond her 3 years, and she makes my heartbeat flip every day. Her love gets my feet to take off with ease. With her, everything is possible!

You were a young, first-time mum when your child got sick. Probably, lots of your expectations of your baby's early months went out the window. Can you say anything about that?

I grieved for a long time, and still do today, that all parental leave (in Sweden the maternal/paternal leave is 18 months) was used to struggle for our daughter's life. Other mothers met at the open pre-school, had coffee in the park, traveled, fed their children with porridge and purees, struggling with sleepless nights, etc. We were isolated in a room at the children's cancer ward. It felt like we were struggling between life and death, not knowing which way we would fall. It felt like my heart had a thousand holes that constantly oozed blood. But while everything was sad and incredibly heavy, we had the world's finest days according to our conditions. Every day with Estelle felt like the most beautiful, and it is nice to look back on.

Tell me anything else you think might be important.

I would like to highlight the importance of family and friends' support. Dare to contact/call, dare to show that you care and are thinking of the family. Just a text message every now and then, or come by with a lunch box. Why not send a postcard to the department? Do not be afraid to interfere, but expect no answer. Do not ever stop showing your concern!

Hugs,
Amanda

My Notes

CHAPTER FOURTEEN

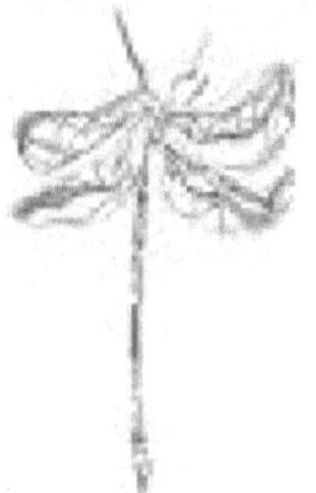

What Are We Going To Do With It?

"If I fail, I try again, and again, and again. If YOU fail, are you going to try again? The human spirit can handle much worse than we realize. It matters HOW you are going to FINISH. Are you going to finish strong?"

— Nick Vujicic

We are now in the long, watchful state of recovery. We are past the chemo, but still dealing with the possibility of after-effects *from* chemo. Yousef's treatments are over, but he still has frequent checkups, tests, and scans to see that the cancer stays away. We are past surgery, but we still have to worry about Yousef's leg, which will never grow on its own. It can only be lengthened so far mechanically -- and then what? We will face that when the time comes.

The life we have now has been shaped by our cancer experience. Whatever adjustments we make every day are just a part of who we are and what we do now. Whatever new strength, awareness, and determination come from that place too. We are stronger than when the cancer interrupted our life because now we look at everything differently.

Like us, you can get through and see your life differently. You don't need to be fearful, bitter or broken. I promise, you have the power to choose how to handle whatever the diagnosis brings, and you *can* guide your child through this. It won't be easy, but you have everything you need to handle it. And if you don't feel so strong all the time, then do not hesitate for a moment to ask for the help you need.

I have always been a positive person, and throughout this whole ordeal, I decided crying wouldn't help anyone. I was determined to be the best possible support for my son. Of course, there were times I did cry, but not in front of Yousef. There were times when I was so afraid, confused, and frustrated – even with my child, who would sometimes resist the medicines or injections I would have to give him. In those raw times, I knew I had to step away so that I could be a help and support to him and not let my emotions run away with me.

I'm sure I didn't do everything right. Neither will you. There is so much parents need to know in order to talk to a child about scary and complicated diagnoses and protocols. You will hear A LOT of information in a short period of time – too much to understand. You will have a hundred questions and not be clear on the answers. You need to weed all that out to make decisions and then tell your child what he or she needs to know. It's OK to make mistakes, to feel like you don't know what you are doing. You can and will figure it out. Be gentle with yourself. One of the physiotherapists at Astrid Lindgren wrote about how important parental support is – and how strong the kids are!

Emilie wrote,

"Working...with children with cancer is difficult but also incredibly rewarding. It is a complex disease, and what is good to do one day may not work at all the day after depending on how the children are doing...the progress is not linear. It is because of the highs and the lows that the child needs more responsiveness from parents and caregivers. But, what I am struck by constantly is how strong the little superheroes are, and how they often will find their own strategies to solve the challenges that we adults never thought about!"

My own little superhero did better than me some days! He handled so much with such courage – and he still does. Someone asked him, "What would you tell another kid who had to go through what you did?"

"I would say, there are days that are really tough and shitty, but there are days that are really fun. Enjoy the time you have and don't think about the negative."

Maybe that sounds more profound coming from him than me! But, I've found there is always something good to notice, even though you might have to look quite hard to find it some days.

Early on in all of this, I decided I would try to grow from what we were going through. It might sound crazy considering how much fear and uncertainty there was. But, we are all tested sometimes, and in the test, is the chance to dig deep inside yourself and grow – to decide who you are. What might you discover about yourself or your child?

What we think about is so important, and yet, so many thoughts are anxious reactions to what goes on around us. Yes, bad things happen, our kids get sick. And, the question is, what are we going to do with it?

I also decided to "pay it forward," and that's what this book is about. I hope to make donations from its proceeds, and I want to help other families going through the same thing we did. This book is not necessarily just for parents, but other people dealing with cancer, or the problems of illness, the medical system, or coping with life and death issues. Yousef is already asking about my next book, too!

I rely on questions – they are the foundation of my life. Questions empower us, and thinking we have all the answers disempowers. That's when we stop looking for miracles and opportunities. Being in the question, never claiming to know the answer, that's where the possibilities are.

A question can change the energy of any situation you find yourself in. Being willing to continually ask will open the door to a whole different life. Whenever something challenged me, I would ask, "What else is possible now?" As I tried my best to get through the past three years, I must have asked it a thousand times, for a thousand different reasons.

Thoughts are reactions to what goes on around us. I've learned not to believe the first thought, but to ask a question and see if the thought can be changed to something positive. Yousef seems to have learned that, too!

I am grateful - I am sure that sounds strange to some people. But through this experience, I learned to take nothing for granted and to live in the NOW. We could be taken away from each other at any moment, so we have to be there for each other and for ourselves. I have the gift of more time with Yousef. Who knows how long any of us have with our children? Don't wait for someone to get sick to begin to appreciate the time. Don't wait for anything.

I would tell a parent going through what I went through to remember all of your children need you, even as you have to devote yourself to the one who is sick. I had to be there for all my children, and so will you. During this time, my eldest daughter had just gotten married, and my younger daughter was finishing University. My older son was applying to go to University. They all needed my support, too. I am proud of all of them – how they were there for their brother, and each contributed what he or she could.

I am the mother of four. I've always put everyone else before me. I've learned how important it is to take care of myself, now. I think about the salt baths I took in Germany, in the privacy of my hotel room. They were more than a retreat – they were healing, a chance to stop thinking, to switch off. Through our time in hospitals, I didn't always have this luxury, but I'd tell you to take every opportunity you can to nurture yourself.

The late Louise Hay said that it is so important that parents love themselves first. She believed if we all did, it would be a much more loving world. We'd be not only caring for our kids differently, we'd be teaching them – modeling for them - self-care and self-love, too.

Let me take some of the guilt away. Caring for yourself is not selfish. It is necessary. Let me also tell the parent who has to keep working not to feel guilty. You can't be everywhere at once. Play your part to the best of your ability.

Probably, the sort of cancer your child has is different from Yousef's. Maybe he or she is older or younger than Yousef was. Maybe different things complicated your life or got in the way of your child's treatment. But many of the same things are true: you must take care of yourself, stay in the present, breathe, look for the beautiful and the positive, and find the love.

It has become so clear to me how much more research is still needed for children's cancer. Here in Sweden, the Childhood Cancer Foundation's goal is to eradicate cancer, but as I see it, it really needs to be a worldwide effort.

I have become very aware of the need for aftercare – support for the family once the child is released from the hospital, told to go home and take the treatments prescribed, and get the child in school again and begin life over. After all the support of round-the-clock nursing care, it is scary to bring home a child and know it's only you now. After being a part of a protocol that tells you exactly what to do if something medical comes up with your child, now we have to explain how he is a cancer survivor to every doctor or dentist we see. Some won't treat him for the most basic things, because now, postcancer, things are complicated – and maybe they fear doing something wrong. I imagine having to explain the diagnosis and treatment over and over until Yousef is old enough to tell himself whenever he needs a routine booster shot for this or an ordinary prescription for that.

My goal with this book was to give some hope and comfort from my own family's experience. I want you to know there is an end, though you may not see it yet, and I don't know what it is for you. The first thought most parents have is that their child will die. But know that there are so many survivors, more and more every year. So rather than sink in fear, believe your child will be one of the survivors. And to keep doing that, you must do everything in your power to remember that your thoughts are just thoughts.

Bless you and your family as you go through an ordeal you could neither prepare for nor anticipate. Know you are not alone, and may you look for blessings along the way.

My Notes

Afterword: Now

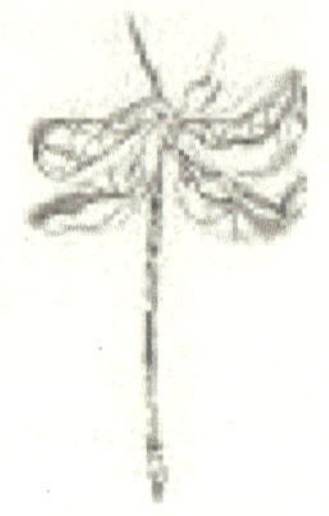

You cannot go back.
But,
Who you are doesn't
end. You are different –
He is different.
"Look how I run!" my 11-year-old starting-over child calls to me.
Look how he has learned.
To run.
Regardless that he has lived in his body and learned these things before.
This is your child too. Or will be.
She may have to learn how to speak, how to see, how to move. She, like a baby, starts to walk and learn new things – because now she is a different person.
We are a different family.
And so are you.
I cheer on my starting-over child. I watch him run.
You will not be the same.
But you will have so much more.
Than before.
You are not alone.

Using the Power of Questions

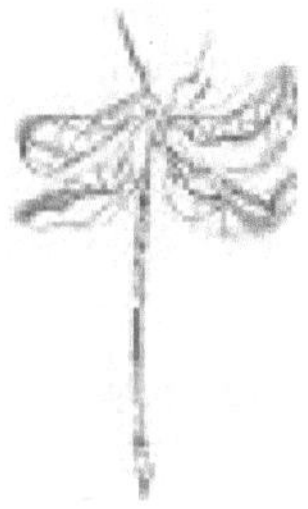

If there is a tough choice, time or place, ask:

What can I do to change this for the greater?

What else is possible here?

What is this?

What can I do with this?

Can I change it?

How do I change it?

If I was to choose what's true for me, what would I be choosing?

What's right about this?

What am I good at that will be easy for me and helpful now?

What awareness do I have here?
What else might I choose to feel right now?

www.ingramcontent.com/pod-product-compliance
Lightning Source LLC
LaVergne TN
LVHW041113150826
845673LV00007B/2035
* 9 7 9 8 7 7 5 8 0 2 9 2 9 *